THE SUCCESSFUL

TREATMENT OF

BRAIN CHEMICAL IMBALANCE

THE SUCCESSFUL
TREATMENT OF
BRAIN CHEMICAL IMBALANCE

By Feel Right, Inc., written by Martin T. Jensen, M.D.
Adult and Child Psychiatrist
Foreword by Lani O'Grady

KENDALL/HUNT PUBLISHING COMPANY
4050 Westmark Drive   Dubuque, Iowa 52002

For additional copies of this manual:

Please call toll-free 1-800-228-0810 or fax 1-800-772-9165
International 1-319-589-1000 or fax 1-319-589-1046

Kendall/Hunt Customer Service
Kendall/Hunt Publishing Company
4050 Westmark Drive, P.O. Box 1840
Dubuque, IA 52004-1840

For appointments or telephone consultations with Dr. Jensen,
please call 714-457-8785.

Table of Contents

BRAIN
CHEMICAL
IMBALANCE
Martin T. Jensen, M.D.
Adult & Child Psychiatry

It is a physician's privilege to have treatment latitude to follow the method outlined in this book if it appears there is merit. This method has not been scientifically tested. What can be said however, is that is has helped thousands of patients get well, including actress Lani O'Grady. After being treated by 32 doctors, and having their techniques fail, this method got her well.

Artwork by Dr. Martin Jensen

Foreword
By Lani O'Grady

Have you ever had feelings of panic, anxiety, depression, anger, frustration, rage, thoughts of suicide or hurting someone? Are you currently taking medication that isn't working? Are you using alcohol or drugs to hide from the awful way you feel? Have you ever wondered why you feel the way you do?

Perhaps the doctor or doctors you're seeing can't seem to find what will help you feel better. Are you tired of hearing "it's all in your head" or "just a little more therapy about what happened to you as a child and you should feel better?" The one I used to hear the most was "if only you could get angry enough at your parents, and vent this frustration, then all your panic, anxiety, depression, abuse of prescription pills, and alcohol would simply go away!" Maybe you have a character trait you would like to change, such as tension, temper, inability to concentrate or disorganization. Are you tired a lot of the time and unable to get enough sleep? Do you eat too little or too much? All of these questions and their solutions are contained in this manual.

For over 20 years of my life, I suffered from panic, anxiety, agoraphobia, and abuse of alcohol and drugs. I had been to a total of 32 doctors over 18 years—from psychiatrists to psychologists, internists, G.P.'s, neurologists, gynecologists, herb doctors, acupuncturists. You name it, I saw one. The only kind of doctor I didn't see was a vet!

Then one day I was recommended to a psychiatrist (a type of doctor I had come to dislike immensely) who I was told practiced a bit differently than most. Because of his success, he was Associate Medical Director of a hospital and had a very busy practice. I made an appointment with this 33rd doctor. He tried medication which other doctors had not tried on me. This doctor did not believe in keeping me on medication that wasn't working for 6-8 weeks. I was desperate and sick and tired of being sick and tired. Even after 5 years of sobriety in the past, it was simply not enough.

The first appointment was only the beginning of what I was soon to learn was the most unique and logical way to approach fixing my problem. Here was a doctor who, rather than treating the symptoms (the panic, anxiety, and abuse), treated the problem: the chemicals in my brain. I was soon to learn that once the brain chemistry was stabilized, and all was normalized inside, all, and I mean ALL of my symptoms went away.

The day Dr. Jensen figured out which medication was going to be the right one, I was well within one hour. I took several medications before he figured out exactly which part of my brain was in crisis, but for every reaction I had from each medication, he seemed to learn more. He was like a chemist and a scientist who was also a psychiatrist. He understood the chemistry of the brain so well, that it was almost mathematical to him. This man knew what he was doing, and the day I got well was a day I had waited

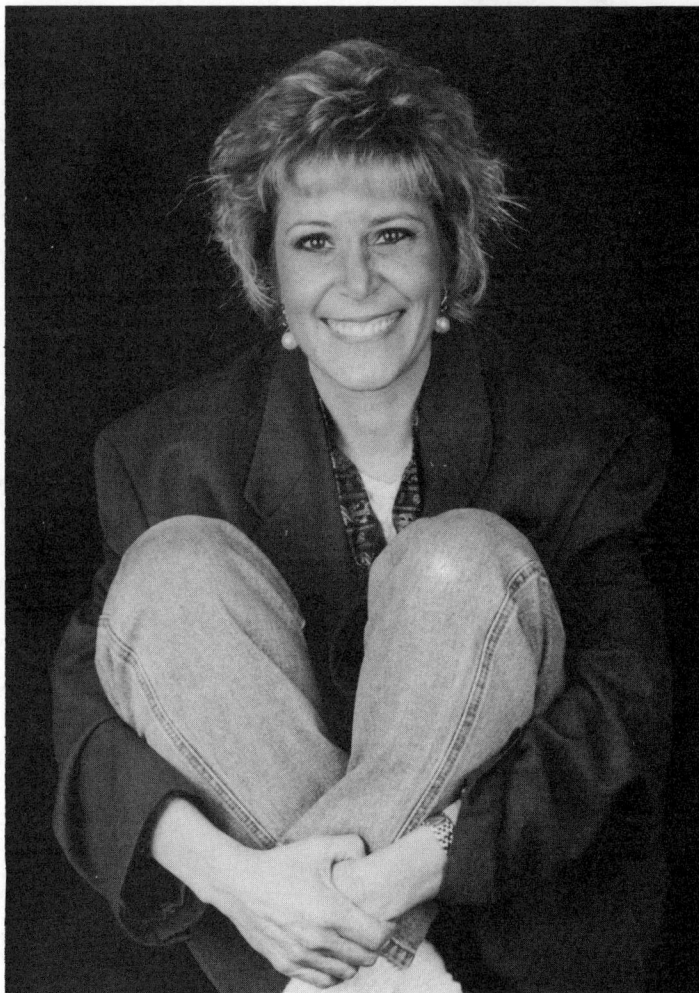

for forever.

This manual is about hope! It is meant to be used as a guide and a tool. Hopefully a physician you have a rapport with will be open to trying new ways to help you feel better. There is one thing very important I want you to understand. We didn't get sick overnight, and we do not usually get well overnight, either. I didn't give up and neither did Dr. Jensen. That's what it takes to get well if you have a brain chemical imbalance: Persistence. The ones who do not get well from this method are primarily those who are too afraid to take medication, and continue the process. It sure feels good to know I wasn't going crazy all those years, and that there was a cure out there, and a way of figuring out what was making me suffer.

I do believe in most standard medical practices. However if you are anything like me, no other method helped, and you are at the point where you don't like the quality of your life. I believe this book can help you change that.

The information contained in this manual, can answer questions you have never received answers for, and can give you hope and inspiration to continue trying to get well. Whatever you do, you cannot give up. There is a doctor somewhere near you that can work through this with you. Doctors are anxious to help their patients feel better and, if there is some information in this manual that can help them do that, most of them will be willing to use this as a tool to help you feel "normal."

Now, as I am currently working in Dr. Jensen's office, I am enjoying on a daily basis watching other people get well from a variety of problems. It feels good to be even a small part of helping them to get better.

I wish you luck. I wish you strength to continue your personal struggle, and hope for you what I got from this type of medical treatment: that you get well.

In a book that is for patients as well as doctors, it is inevitable that words and concepts will be read that cannot be understood. Relax, check the glossary, and ask your doctor for further explanations.

Fondly,

Lani O'Grady

LANI O'GRADY
"Eight is Enough"
MARY BRADFORD

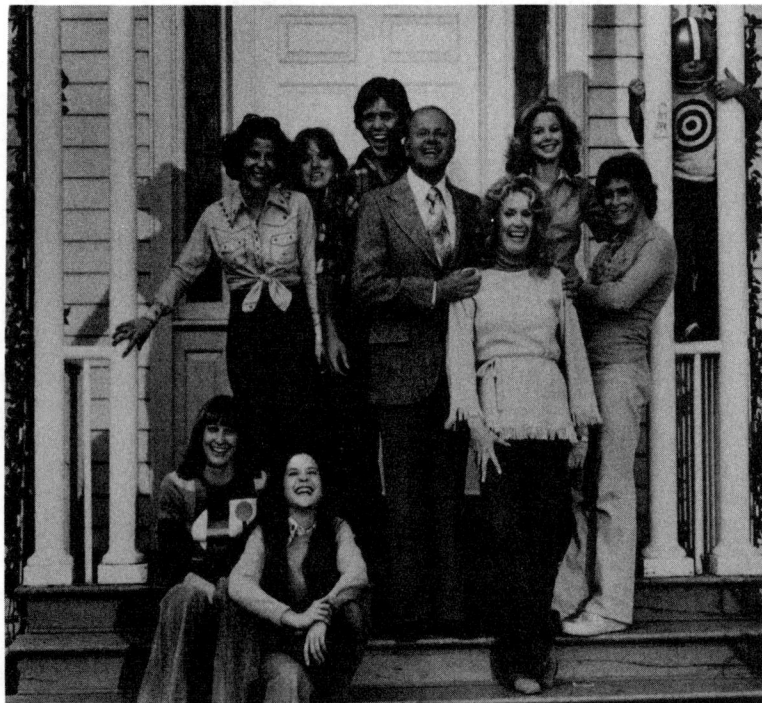

"Eight is Enough"

CHAPTER 1

INTRODUCTION TO BRAIN NORMALIZATION

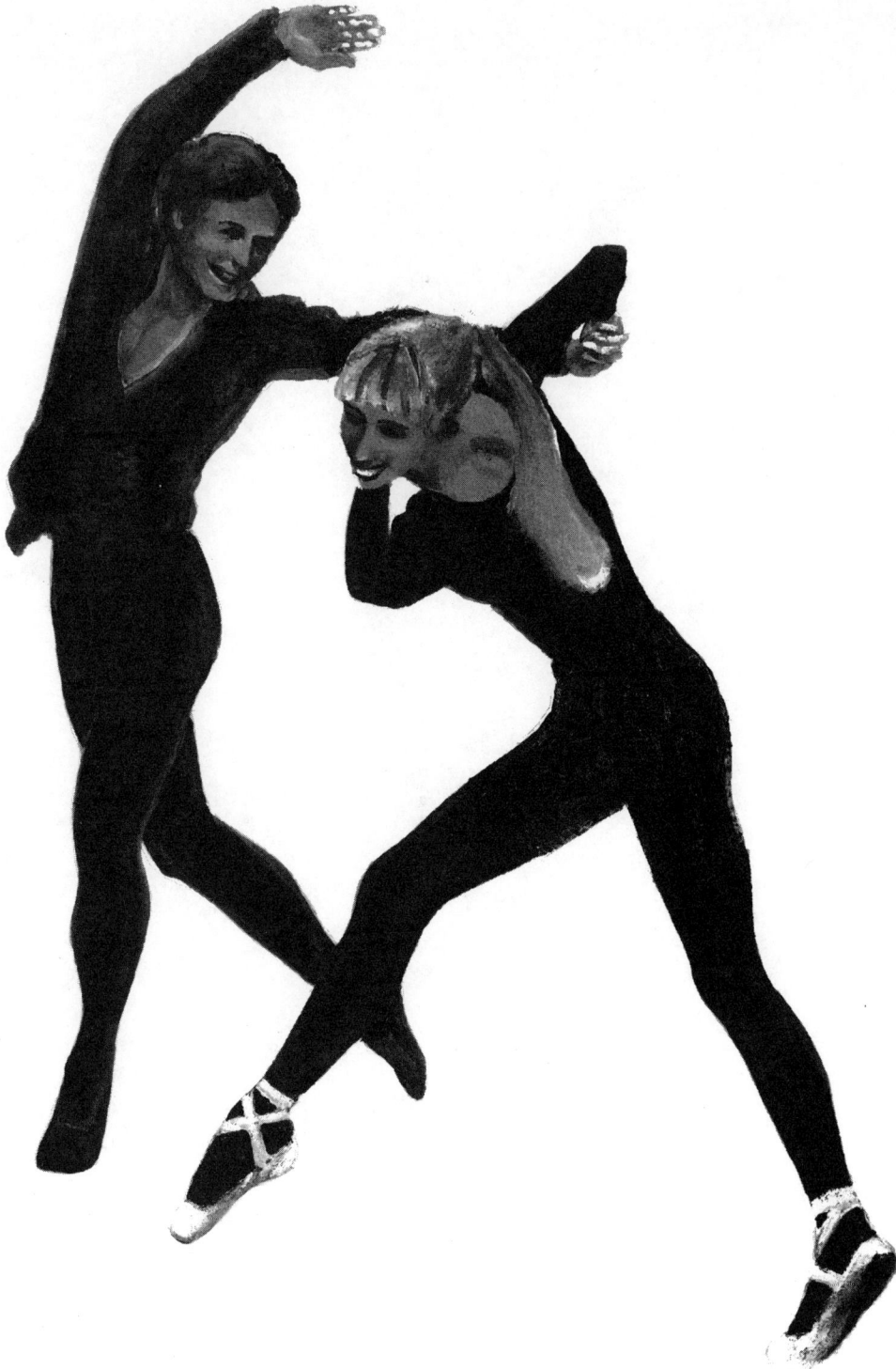

BRAIN NORMALIZATION
An Introduction

What is a Chemical Imbalance?

Everyone has chemical differences in their brain. Sometimes this is an asset and other times a handicap. If it is causing a problem with the quality of your life, it is worth treating. Stress can temporarily amplify these differences. A true chemical imbalance is when a physical problem causes psychological signs and the person doesn't get to feel normal. The brain is supposed to make several different chemicals. If one is missing, low or excessive, it can cause behavioral changes and discomfort of many types.

How Can You Tell if You Have a Chemical Imbalance?

You may have feelings or behavior unacceptable to yourself or others. You may have recurrent feelings of depression, anxiety, or a decrease in your level of functioning that cannot be explained or solved by traditional treatment methods, such as support groups or psychotherapy. In short, you don't feel right, reality doesn't explain the feelings or behavior, and it keeps on happening. Some chemical imbalances may not be compatible with life. Blood testing is often a part of the initial evaluation, but usually more is learned from the personal and family history, and reactions to past medications. If you have a genetic background of volatility, you are not at fault for it. You inherited it. But, you can fix it. Your ancestors had no choice, you do. Now the chemical workhorse in your brain that is not working can be identified.

How Do People Cope?

Most patients with a chemical imbalance have been told it is all "in their head." Usually these patients have been from doctor to doctor seeking relief only to be subjected to extensive and expensive lab tests which, often show nothing abnormal. Completely frustrated, current as well as past generations have sought comfort in destructive methods: alcohol, drug abuse, sex, violence and suicide. The problem with these solutions is they only provide temporary relief from the symptoms of the chemical imbalance, but do nothing to correct the problem. The solution may cause further deterioration, or even death. It is hard enough dealing with the world, without having to fight your own brain chemistry. Some chemical imbalances are terrorizing and unrelenting. Others are brief and related to a crisis. Medical comfort is usually possible for either situation, on a temporary or long term basis.

How Do You Find Relief?

The answer is really amazingly simple. There are ten systems in the brain. Through a series of steps, the system that isn't working can be readily identified and corrected. First, the doctor must rule out disease as the cause of the patient's symptoms. This, of course, is done through physical examination and lab tests. Most of my patients usually arrive in my office with long histories of laboratory tests and physical exams done to determine the cause of their distress.

The initial interview explores the clinical history using the intake form found on page 34 of this manual. The history of adverse reactions to various medicines and substances provides "clues" to the malfunctioning system and is recorded on the medication worksheet on page 37. This is different from the typical patient history done in most doctor's offices. It is designed to analyze the ten systems, find "clues" to the malfunctioning system and narrow the choices.

This initial interview will usually allow the doctor to narrow the possible causes from 10 to 2 or 3. The signs are often there. Next, based on the "clues," a protocol is prescribed. A protocol consists of three different medications, each designed to address one of the "clues" discovered through the interview.

For example, based on the symptoms charted during the initial interview, a patient suffering from severe anxiety might be prescribed an antidepressant to address low serotonin, a mood stabilizer to reduce norepinephrine instability and an anticonvulsant to address possible electrical instability — each a pos-

11

sible cause of the anxiety. Patients who have not tried any of these medicines usually follow the protocols which are in chapter 3. This covers most brain chemistry types within 5 visits.

Each medication is prescribed in "sample doses" — no more than five to seven days worth of each and taken one at a time. Specific instructions are written for each medication along with an antidote to relieve unwelcome side affects which may occur if the medication isn't hitting the target. This "sampling" gives the patient the ability to quickly test a possible remedy without having to wait four to six weeks to see if it works. When only a few medicines were invented, it was important to wait 6 weeks for a "domino effect" to occur. Now that there are many medicines, it is usually more advantageous to briefly compare them first to find an exact match that works the same day. The farther a cure is from the problem, the longer it takes to work if it works at all. The right medication usually works the same day and the patient will know it. This is the basis of the success I've had with my patients.

A follow-up appointment occurs two to three weeks from the initial visit. By this time, the patient has tested each of the three medications and can report the results. Sometimes one of the medications hits the target immediately and the patient returns to report its success. Other times it takes several tries to further narrow the possible causes, get the right medication and the right dosage. But rarely does it take longer.

Why Medications?

The use of medication has become quite common yet sometimes controversial in the treatment of chemical imbalance. However, many people are deciding they do not have to suffer while solving life's problems. Some people are so affected and uncomfortable that they cannot even respond to conventional therapy until they normalize their chemistry. Others appreciate learning and "typing-out" their chemistry so they can use a safe anti-stress pill temporarily in times of crisis, until it has blown over. Most people use these medications to help during a difficult period of their life.

You have a right to control your own brain, and not have it controlling you. These protocols also give patients responsibility for their recovery as well as control, something they seem to appreciate. By allowing them to "test" a medication and retain or discard it based on its success, a patient derives a sense of ownership in his/her recovery and a sense of control — something usually left in the hands of the doctor.

It is a Quality of Life Decision

An emerging trend is that people often choose to check out their genetic background (what traits and characteristics they were born with) before spending years in therapy. Of course, counseling for stress and social adjustment can help anyone, but when symptoms are debilitating or destructive, medication is indicated. Leaving the brain chemistry uncorrected can cause distress and unnecessary suffering for you and your loved ones. There is a general awareness of statistics concerning addiction, suicide, and violence in America, and they are frightening. Exploring family backgrounds often reveals shocking casualty rates of drinking, depression, panic disorder or other dysfunction. Technology has caught up with this so the suffering can now stop. Victims in silent anguish no longer have to continue to hurt.

I believe we are entering the era of the brain. America's pain is mental. The good news is that most chemical imbalances are curable. It is wonderful that a modern attitude is replacing outdated embarrassment, shame and guilt. People are getting well. Correcting chemical imbalances can unlock and clear family tensions. Life no longer has to be so hard. For the first time in human history, everyone has the privilege and right to have their brain transmitters operating normally.

How My Method Evolved

I graduated from Oklahoma College of Medicine in 1980, and from an adult and child psychiatry residency (Medical College of Pennsylvania) in 1985. From the onset I did not completely trust the simple concept that a given mental illness had only one cure. I vaguely believed that any mental complaint probably had a variety of causes.

In 1986, while treating hyperactive school children, a 29-year old female patient who had been hospitalized since her teens because of suicide attempts, bulimia and anxiety requested help from me. She had been on every category of medicine except Ritalin. I wondered if she had the equivalent chemistry of a hyperactive child, even though she could concentrate and had never been hyperactive. I felt this patient had nothing to lose so gave her, in the hospital, a child's dose of Ritalin. Within one hour she felt completely normal. She was released from the hospital and never set foot in one again. She enrolled in a small college, became valedictorian, and eventually became a social worker. This is now 1995 and she continues to visit my office every 6 months for a 12% child's dose of Ritalin.

After this experience, I made sure that any patient not getting well tried all categories of mental medicines. Then came a second surprise. I took care of severely ill and often "resistant" patients, and approximately one-third of them got well on medications that did not match their diagnosis. I then gradually came to realize that each of standard psychiatry's 370 diagnoses, for the most part, had 9 possible causes for men and 10 for women.

Then the bad news about Prozac started. It was feared that Prozac possibly caused mental worsening and suicide. However, I observed that these Prozac victims were actually normal appearing people with hidden threads of manic depressive, psychotic or attention deficit disorder chemistry (see next chapter). They could not be diagnosed "by the book" because they looked only depressed. Furthermore, as I learned, any antidepressant, not just Prozac, could induce problems in these patients.

A reliable antidote, dopamine reduction, was found for all antidepressant destabilizations. I realized then that these adverse antidepressant reactions could be used diagnostically to define underlying brain chemistry.

The **medication reactions became more reliable than the clinical picture in guiding treatment** and I actively sought to understand adverse medication reactions from all 9-10 categories, and establish antidotes for these.

Many treatment-resistant patients have improved with this method. For example, a man who had seen over 100 doctors was fixed in one visit (see page 22). Then Lani came through my practice and got well using this method after 32 other physicians had failed her. Next, publicity occurred. People began to seek the same results so I converted the above, which was mostly intuitive, into a concrete diagnostic procedure: **a check list for 10 systems in the brain**. Close observation, statistics (chapter 4), and perseverance were the final ingredients improving treatment success.

This method relies on medication reactions to guide treatment. It is given a framework by an aggressive five part plan which tests nine to ten types of brain chemistry, in such a way that the disturbed system(s) can be identified and corrected.

This approach opens the doors to treatment for many people. One thing that has interferred with people seeking or getting treatment is a worry of being negatively labeled. For example, would you rather be diagnosed as having "moodiness" due to unstable electricity (fixable in 2 hours), or be labeled manic depressive? Would you prefer to have a mild 3% dopamine ("DA") elevation causing insomnia, or be told you have psychotic features? These new terms are medical, kinder, and roughly more accurate. They are "user friendly" words that make treatment less stigmatic. The chemical labels also result in greater nonprejudicial fluidity of treatment for the spectrum of chemical imbalances.

BRAIN
CHEMICAL
IMBALANCE
Martin T. Jensen, M.D.
Adult & Child Psychiatry

How To Use This Manual

This manual was written for both patient and doctor. The first four chapters are an overview of the disorders commonly found in patients, my method for narrowing the "clues," the protocols prescribed for the "clues," samples of forms used during treatment, and statistical proof of the success of these methods from my practice. By the time you've completed this section, hopefully you will have an understanding of what needs to be done.

It is my hope that, if you are a person suffering from an unknown and unsuccessfully treated ailment, you might share this manual with your doctor and ask that he/she explore with you its contents. Together, you can find the help you've been looking for.

Chapters 5 through 10 are designed for the medical professional. However, if you're the patient and wish to try your hand at understanding the technical jargon of our profession, feel free to dive in. They are designed to help the medical professional understand where conventional psychiatric therapy and my techniques blend.

Summation

One patient described how a doctor, trying to find the cause of her anxiety disorder, told her "you have reached the end of the medical model." That is because several types of brain chemistry are not clinically recognizable on the surface. Looking at medication reactions (biological markers) and statistics in the framework of medication protocols, allows us to identify these patients so treatment can be successful. This patient got well in two visits using the method in Chapter 3.

As you solve your chemical imbalance with your doctor, it is your doctor who will ultimately decide and weigh risks. The elderly, the medically compromised, pregnant or nursing women, children, and chemically dependent and addicted patients require special consideration concerning medication selection and dosage. Your doctor should be alerted to any of the above risk factors.

This book is a description of the successful work I do. It is the result of ten years of clinical observation, perseverance and success. It "dives" into brain chemistry. This is my method. It has not been scientifically tested as superior to standard treatment. However, because of the success I've seen with this method, people throughout the country have asked that I write down what I do and how. This manual is meant only to do that. Hopefully, if you're one of the millions of people who suffer from a chemical imbalance, this book will be useful to you and your doctor as you work together to find the cause and the cure.

The brain is a universe. I hope you will, if necessary, explore the boundaries of your chemistry. I wish you the best of luck in successfully solving the imbalance and attaining the normal, happy productive life that can be yours.

COMMON CHEMICAL IMBALANCES

CHAPTER 2

1 - Serotonin Low
2 - Norepinephrine Low
3 - Chemistry Unstable
4 - Electricity Unstable
5 - Dopamine High
6 - Chemistry Failed
7 - Gaba Malfunctioning
8 - Adrenaline High
9 - Thyroid Malfunction
10 - Estrogen Low
(Females)

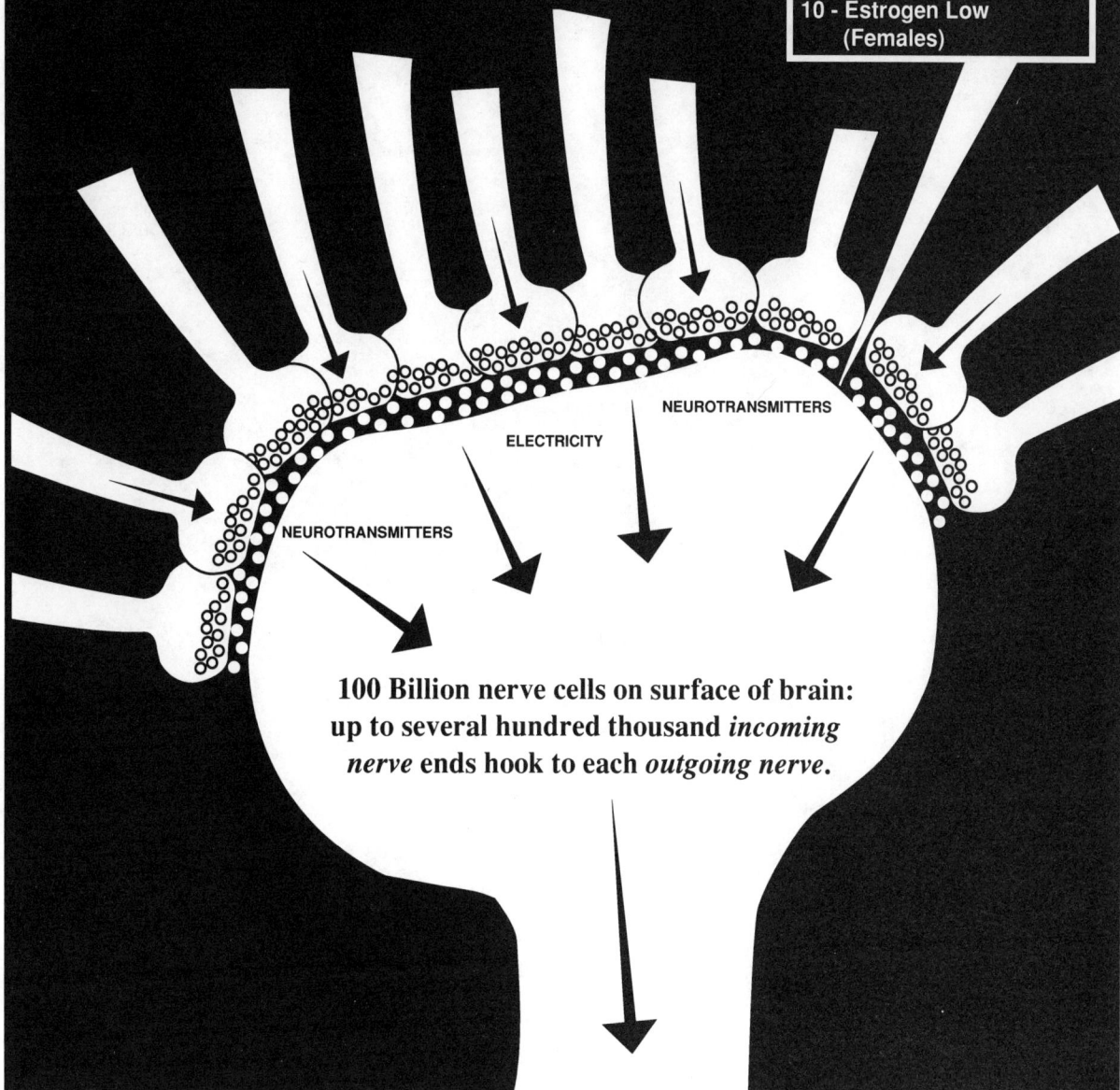

NEUROTRANSMITTERS

ELECTRICITY

NEUROTRANSMITTERS

100 Billion nerve cells on surface of brain: up to several hundred thousand *incoming* nerve ends hook to each *outgoing* nerve.

TEN COMMON IMBALANCES
Their Chemical Names

There are 10 systems (9 in men) that can be the cause of most symptoms of an imbalance.

1. Low Serotonin (SE)

2. Low Noreprinephrine (NE)

3. Unstable Chemicals (NE, SE)

4. Unstable Electricity

5. High Dopamine (DA)

6. Failed Chemicals (DA/NE)

7. Malfunctioning GABA

8. High Adrenaline

9. Malfunctioning Thyroid

10. Low Estrogen (women only)

On the first visit to my office, I conduct a thorough interview of the patient's clinical and medical history using the patient intake form and medication worksheet on page 34 and 37. This is done in conjunction with a recent physical exam and laboratory testing. Depending on the symptoms I may order a free T4, FTI and TSH, SMA25, CBC, VDRL, and UA. Based on the results of this initial screen, more specialized tests are ordered to identify any physical factors.

SIX GENERAL PRESENTATIONS OF ILLNESS

Most complaints fall into one of the following six clinical categories. These categories are, in my opinion, especially useful in treatment.

Many patients, however, do not fall into only one category but, may have a small component from one or more of the categories.

Each of these categories has any of 10 types of chemistry as its cause. The graphs in Chapter 4 (Statistics from My Practice) show how fixing these chemistries will fix most mental conditions.

■ **ANXIETY** (Other related conditions include panic disorder, agoraphobia, and social phobia). Victims of panic may experience shortness of breath, palpitations, dizziness, trembling, sweating, nausea, numbness, confusion, fear of dying, and even chest pain. Agoraphobia also includes a fear of being in places from which escape is difficult (crowds, lines, traffic, airplanes, etc.). Anxiety disorders are the most prevalent cause of emotional suffering in America.

Classically low GABA, low serotonin and low NE are treated. My observations indicate anxiety disorders can be subtyped according to which neurotransmitter abnormality is present. Low serotonin/NE (48%); GABA (24%); chemical instability (22%); chemical failure (14%); electrical instability (14%); or high DA (13%). Thyroid dysfunction factors are in 24%.

■ **DEPRESSION** is characterized by sadness, insomnia (or excess sleep), fatigue, weight loss or gain, irritability, feelings of worthlessness, decreased concentration and thoughts of death. Medication can often comfort this within hours, but sometimes in several weeks.

Classically the chemistry is low serotonin and/or low NE (47%). My observations indicate also that chemical instability (29%); GABA malfunction (15%); electricial instability (14%); dopamine elevaton (13%); chemical failure (12%); thyroid dysfunction factors (28%); or any compromised system can cause depression.

■ **MANIC DEPRESSION** (also known as **bipolar** disorder) is characterized sometimes by talkativeness and irritability. These patients can act sexually aroused, grandiose, confident and expansive. The severe mood instability can be recurring euphoria or irritability alternating with intense depression. Other symptoms may include decreased sleep, high energy, agitation, and reckless judgement (buying sprees, impulsive or unwise sex, foolish driving, etc.).

The chemistry is chemical or electrical instability. Other disorders can resemble this classic diagnosis. Seasonal affective disorder is often associated with "manic depressive" chemistry. See graph on page 84.

■ **SCHIZOPHRENIA (psychosis)** is characterized by hallucinations, incoherence, delusions, bizarreness, loss of social behavior and general functioning. The brain transmitter dopamine, depending on the degree of elevation, can cause mild to severe symptoms in this direction. Organic syndromes and manic depression can also cause psychosis.

> *The chemistry is dopamine elevation in 65%. Low serotonin/NE can resemble this in 27%; chemical instability (18%); GABA (18%); electrical instability (6%); or chemical failure (3%). Thyroid dysfunction may be present in 21%.*

■ **ATTENTION-DEFICIT HYPERACTIVITY DISORDER (ADHD)** is usually characterized by inattentiveness, difficulty concentrating, over-activity (especially in childhood), fidgeting, inability to stay with a task, excessive talking, and possibly thrill seeking. In 70% of children with ADHD, this persists into adulthood because their nervous system fails to mature.
ATTENTION DEFICIT DISORDER (ADD) is essentially the same, but without the hyperactivity.

> *The chemistry is chemical failure causing low blood flow to several areas of the brain. Similar symptoms can occur from chemical or electrical instability and dopamine elevation. Abnormal thyroid genetics 38% of the time can also cause this as an injury or is associated with this chemistry.*

■ **ORGANIC SYNDROMES** include Alzheimers, various medical injuries (stroke), and conditions (for example, thyroid disturbance, drug and alcohol intoxication and withdrawal). Numerous causes exist including especially aging, seizures, amphetamine abuse, prolonged alcoholism and AID's. Thinking and social judgement can be impaired, and personality changed. Sometimes memory is deficient. In severe cases, disorientation, incoherence and psychosis occur. Occasionally mood is the only altered feature.

> *Any of the ten types of brain chemistry can be affected, yet typically electrical instability, dopamine elevation or chemical failure is the problem. Thyroid malfunction genetics are a common cause of these injuries. Alcohol is probably poor quality liquid GABA and is commonly abused to anesthetize other brain transmitter problems. Estrogen failure (for example, menopause) can cause dopamine elevation distress.*

Chemical imbalance can be "masked."

Childhood chemical imbalance may be evidenced by stomach aches, isolation, anxiety, misbehavior or defiance. *Teenage* chemical imbalance may be evidenced by substance abuse, promiscuity, stealing, messy poor hygiene or headaches.

In *adults*, low back pain, heart symptoms, stomach discomforts, and urinary tract problems can be due to or exacerbated by chemical imbalance. Insomnia, fatigue and headaches are common.

In the *elderly,* similar symptoms can occur, but thinking difficulties resembling dementia may be due to chemical imbalance.

TEN MEDICAL CHOICES TO NORMALIZE THE BRAIN
Are All Systems Working?

In standard treatment, after a diagnosis is made, medication is prescribed and tried for a three to six week period for most disorders. If it is working it is continued, if not, another medication is tried or added.

Several major classes of medication have been found to be helpful in treating chemical imbalance. Note that at this time, there are **ten primary access points into the brain's chemistry**, listed below:

Medicine	Systems Effecting the Brain	Illness
Mood Elevators ● Antidepressants	*Raises* 1. Low Serotonin (S) *And/Or* 2. Low Norepinephrine (NE) + Low Dopamine (DA/NE)	Depression
Mood Stabilizers ● Lithium ● Anticonvulsants	*Stabilizes* 3. Chemical Instability 4. Electrical Instability	Manic Depression
Antipsychotics ● Neuroleptics	*Reduces* 5. Elevated Dopamine (DA)	Psychosis
Stimulants ● Amphetamines	*Replaces* 6. Failed Chemical(s) Dopamine/Norepinephrine (DA/NE)	Attention Deficit Disorder
Anxiety Reducers ● Benzodiazepines ● Beta-adrenergic Blockers	*Enhances* 7. "GABA" which inhibits other transmitters 8. Adrenaline blockade	Anxiety Palpitations
Hormonal ● Thyroid ● Estrogen	*Augments* 9. Thyroid Malfunction And Metabolic Rate *Augments* 10. Low Estrogen in Females	Low Thyroid Low Estrogen

References on medication actions can be found on page 190. See Chapter 5 for details on these medications.

If the wrong access point is picked, the medicine may take a long time to work. In fact, it may never work. When large medication doses are required, the access point may be incorrect. **Exact matches usually translate to lower dosages and quick results.** When medication choices were few, a six-week trial period was important. Now that a wide variety of safe new medications are available, it is usually possible to find a match that succeeds within 24 hours.

PUTTING THE CHEMICAL AND CLINICAL TOGETHER
Typical case examples from each category

1. LOW SEROTONIN [S]

A low serotonin perfectionistic personality may exist. This deficiency can be an asset and a handicap. Organized, tense people often have low serotonin. They may be anxious and alcohol prone (1-2 glasses or more per day). Some hypochondriacs have low serotonin, as do many people who suffer emotionally. The family history is often positive for cancer, raising the question if low serotonin compromises the immune system.

•A marine sergeant suffered for decades, as had his father, with **tension** and **temper**. Within hours after serotonin correction (Prozac), he was relaxed and normal. He was astonished and asked "Why didn't I do this 20 years ago?"
    Answer: This was not invented 20 years ago.

•A volatile, suicidal, unstable teenager and her meticulous mother (with hypothyroidism) had low serotonin. Zoloft worked in hours and did not cause worsening as Prozac had. The thyroid genetics apparently contaminated the brain chemistry with instability.

•A **tense**, **perfectionistic, alcohol prone** lawyer after Prozac serotonin enhancement felt much better in hours. His drinking excess normalized to a comfortable one drink per week.

•Two parents, low in serotonin were fixed completely using Paxil. Their eight year old child was **unhappy** and emotionally disturbed. She was given the same medicine as her parents. Within two hours she became normal and free from the inherited genetic curse.

2. LOW NOREPINEPHRINE [NE] [or low DA (dopamine)/NE]

•A **fatigued**, tired, **obese** woman could not stop **binging** and felt very depressed. Norpramine (NE. antidepressant) helped her within 1 day. She then raised the dose and felt better, energetic and no longer pressured to binge. She still had to work hard to lose weight, and did.

•A cocaine addict stopped his habit, but still had strong **cocaine cravings** due to depleted NE. Norpramine helped this, but gradually over a 2 week period.

•A laboratory technician found she had mild dopamine/ norepinephrine failure responsive to Wellbutrin. An adverse reaction to a serotonin agent guided her to this. Before getting the medicine, she complained of being **"scatter-brained"** and **depressed**.

Even though the serotonin and norepinephrine systems feed into each other, patients usually prefer one antidepressant type over another. If any other chemical imbalance (#3 through 10) is present, antidepressants can cause worsening.

3. CHEMICAL INSTABILITY

These people are sometimes **creative, passionate,** and **suicidal.** They can choose drastically idealistic or destructive pursuits, or they can appear as normal.

•An accountant had difficulty organizing thoughts and complained of painful **sensitivity** to rejection, as well as to people in general. His teenage years were dangerously **wild**. Antidepressant adverse reactions guided treatment to lithium, which worked in several hours.

•A teenage, vegetarian honor student with anorexia weighed only 63 lbs. Antidepressant adverse reactions guided treatment to lithium which reversed her downward spiral 3 hours after the first dose. She no longer was suicidal or **emotionally in pain,** and so could eat. Her poetry, art, and music became bright instead of morose.

•A teacher was altruistic, creative and hurting emotionally. A single lithium daily allowed her to feel happy.

•A 79-year old successful entrepreneur had seen over 100 doctors for depression and anxiety. He said substances which stimulated NE (antidepressants, asthma medicines) worsed his condition. After the evaluation, within 2 hours, a single lithium daily allowed him to feel good for the first time in his life, probably for the rest of his life.

My observations suggest chemical instability, like most chemical imbalances can be "patchy" in the brain or body. For example in blood vessels this causes cluster migraine headaches, treatable with lithium. 22% of anxiety disorders are corrected with a small dose of lithium. It is inappropriate to call either of those disorders "manic depression." A "chemical instability" headache or anxiety is more accurate.

4. ELECTRICAL INSTABILITY

DEPAKOTE (divalproex) RESPONSIVE

•A middle-aged woman complained of chronic **moodiness**, **headaches** and **anxiety**. She said all antidepressants worsened her and that lithium didn't help. Electrical smoothing with Depakote made her normal in several hours.

TEGRETAL (carbamazepine) RESPONSIVE

•A **frustrated** middle-aged man who drank when he was younger said he threw and hit things due to a **physical temper**. Antidepressants did not work, nor did lithium. Electrical smoothing with Tegretal made him normal in several hours.

•Some cocaine **damaged**, or heroin **addicted** people find Tegretal helpful in stopping their addictions. They describe that it "mellows" them. Some say Tegretal feels like heroin, even though it is not a narcotic (i.e. it is not addictive, it just smooths electricity).

More Examples

BRAIN
CHEMICAL
IMBALANCE
Martin T. Jensen, M.D.
Adult & Child Psychiatry

5. DOPAMINE ELEVATION [DA]

The classic example of this in severe form is the **schizophrenic** (see chemical imbalance categories description). Milder dopamine elevations occur in "normal people." For example:

• A young woman suffered from **volatility**, and **intensity**. She was unresponsive to other interventions. A 4% dose of Mellaril taken during times of crisis improved her comfort and relaxation levels considerably.

• A young female sober alcoholic had chronic **resistant insomnia**. The only thing to fix this was a 3% dopamine reduction (Mellaril 25mg. at bedtime).

• A patient became **confused** and **hostile**. This was cleared with a 4% dose of Stelazine, and thus she was found to have been 4% dopamine toxic. This stopped working in several months. Further testing (see Protocols in next chapter) revealed DA/NE failure as the primary imbalance. DA/NE replacement (100%) combined with dopamine reduction of 4% provided consistent excellent results.

• A large man **abusing 'crack' cocaine** became **dangerously violent**. Haldol* was given (5mg.) and normalized him.

* Given with Cogentin, a side effect medicine.

My observations suggest that DA elevation can be triggered by extremes of NE or S. For example, cocaine causes high NE. Manic depression causes high or low NE. ADHD is failed NE. Tourettes has low serotonin. All of these in severe form cause DA to increase.

Dopamine is needed in various areas of the brain and body. It makes us walk freely and fluidly, helps orgasm and maintains blood pressure. It is like an amplifier for these functions.

6. CHEMICAL FAILURE [DA/NE] (also called ADD / ADHD)

This is perhaps the most common hidden cause of treatment failure in adults. Symptoms are often vague, severe and confusing. The manual contains protocols which identify and correct this. Also a medication reaction "footprint" may exist and is on page 64.

• A completely **nonfunctional** woman was hospitalized almost continuously for years. She had no symptoms of hyperactivity, and was mainly **agitated, stressed, suicidal** and **alcoholic.** She cleared in 1 hour with a full children's dose of Ritalin.

• A **hyperactive** boy in preschool was starting to **assault** peers. He was about to be expelled permanently. He was medically corrected with a tiny amount of Dexedrine and Clonidine.

Chemical failure can also be "patchy." In one area of the brain this is ADD, another area ADHD, another area narcolepsy and still another area agoraphobia. Stroke phenomena can cause a patch of chemical failure (for example, a cocaine overdose initiating a panic disorder).

More Examples

7. GABA [G] DEFICIENCY

•A woman with much **anxiety** failed to respond at any treaments (antidepressants, mood stabilizers, antipsychotics, ADD medicines). The other medicines usually caused adverse reactions. She felt much better with a GABA agent, and dosage was low enough that tolerance and addiction were unlikely to ever become a problem.

The medical profession may be using this approach (Valium and Xanax) excessively. The mistake is anesthetizing rather than correcting other chemical imbalances. Yet true "low GABA" exists as described above.

GABA's role is to inhibit nerves. It is my observation chemical failure patients (ADHD) may feel worse to have this chemistry inhibited further. Thus an adverse reaction to benzodiazepines (GABA) suggests ADHD.

8. ADRENALINE EXCESS

A woman with hyperthyroidism had panic, pressured speech and heart palpitations. Inderal, a beta blocker helped control the distressing physical symptoms within an hour.

9. THYROID GENETICS (LOW THYROID RESERVOIR)

•A woman with a family history of thyroid problems had normal thyroid test results, but had **fatigue, anxiety,** 40 pounds of **excess weight**, **temperature intolerance** (felt hot), was **losing hair**, and had **brittle nails**. A 5% dose of Cytomel (5mcg.) fixed all this in 3 months. Moods also improved after cytomel was switched to gentler acting synthroid.

The thyroid regulates rate of metabolism for the entire body, and may keep the brain transmitters healthy by keeping neurons stable.

A thyroid difference in the patient, or the patient's family is relevant. The thyroid is the **"wild card"** that can convert normal chemistry into any abnormal chemistry.

Indeed various rat studies indicate that alterations in the thyroid state lead to changes in the norepinephrine (NE) system [reference 26]. My observations indicate on page 58 chemical failure occurs in 38%, low NE or serotonin is in 32% and chemical instability is in 25% of primarily hypothyroid patients.

The prevalence of thyroid abnormalities in attention deficit hyperactivity disorder children ("chemical failure") is greater than 5 times that of the general population. People with a genetic resistance to thyroid hormone have a 46% rate of ADHD [reference 29].

Additional rat studies have demonstrated that decreasing thyroid function lowered brain serotonin [reference 28].Thyroid abnormalities are associated with 50-92% of highly unstable "manic depressive" cases [reference 11, page 357]. Seasonal affective disorder (fall-winter depression) has been linked to manic depression (chemical instability). S.A.D. has low thyroid tests in 35% and borderline low tests in 16% [reference 30].

Schizophrenics (DA overactivity) have reduced thyroid hormone levels compared to healthy subjects [reference 23].

Low thyroid rats show increased sensitivity to dopamine [reference 31].

With this type of data, it is likely that thyroid symptoms or any thyroid family history indicates a likelihood of a genetically different brain.

Unfortunately giving replacement thyroid treatment usually does not fix the wide variety of neurotransmitter "injuries" associated with a thyroid difference. These I identify and neutralize by the method outlined in the next chapter.

10. ESTROGEN DEFICIENCY

Monthly estrogen shots helped a 30 year old female when nothing else worked for her anxiety and depression. Yet some women get worse with estrogen.

Estrogen instability or failure often elevates dopamine 2-3%.

BLENDS

An example of a mixed chemical imbalance is a low serotonin level with slight electrical instability:

 •A bright, but **depressed, nonfunctional** salesman felt better with Paxil, but then in several months destabilized into **hostility** and **forgetfulness**. Adding a 10% dose of electricity smoother (Depakote - 125mg. in the morning daily) resulted in his getting completely well.

Certain blends are difficult, especially when DA/NE failure is occurring since many medicines worsen their symptoms.

CHILDREN

The most common imbalance evident in **children** is **chemical failure** (attention deficit disorder), and occasionally **dopamine excess** (psychosis). For severe anxiety, children have successfully been calmed using low doses of valium.

As a child approaches puberty, all medical approaches to the brain become more relevant.

 •A girl, age 12, was artistic and **emotionally hurting** much of the time. Moods fluctuated between **irritability** and **suicidal thoughts**. A family history revealed **high casualty rates** in parents and grandparents, and suicidal existences. NE. stabilization with a small dose of lithium cleared the girl in one day (150mg. each morning). It is hoped that she was spared the anguish her predecessors experienced.

OLDER ADULTS

In **aging people**, neuronal loss leads especially to GABA deficiency and DA/NE failure, both of which are easily correctable. Confusion may increase due to dopamine elevation: Mellaril 10 - 20mg. at bedtime can help their **insomnia**. Haldol 0.5 - 1mg. per day can also relieve confusion. Though the above patterns are the most common, anything is possible. For this reason, the protocol sequences (next chapter) might best define each persons disability. Medication dosages are usually low.

Studies indicate decreases in DA and NE initiate many declines in bodily funcitons in aging rats and mice [reference 27]. This leads to less thyroid hormone, decreased metabolism, a reduced immune system and more cancer. Chemical failure is due to damage and loss of those neurons. Old rats given drugs that elevate DA/NE experience a reversal or delay of the decrements of aging, and lifespan may be prolonged. DA/NE loss has been reported in humans. [reference 27]

This has been a description of "typical" characteristics of chemical imbalances. However, **the strength of this method is recognizing that most symptoms can be caused by malfunction in any brain transmitter system. For more details see the graphs in Chapter IV for some surprising statistics.**

CHAPTER 3

MY METHOD: TEN MEDICAL SYSTEMS TO CHECK

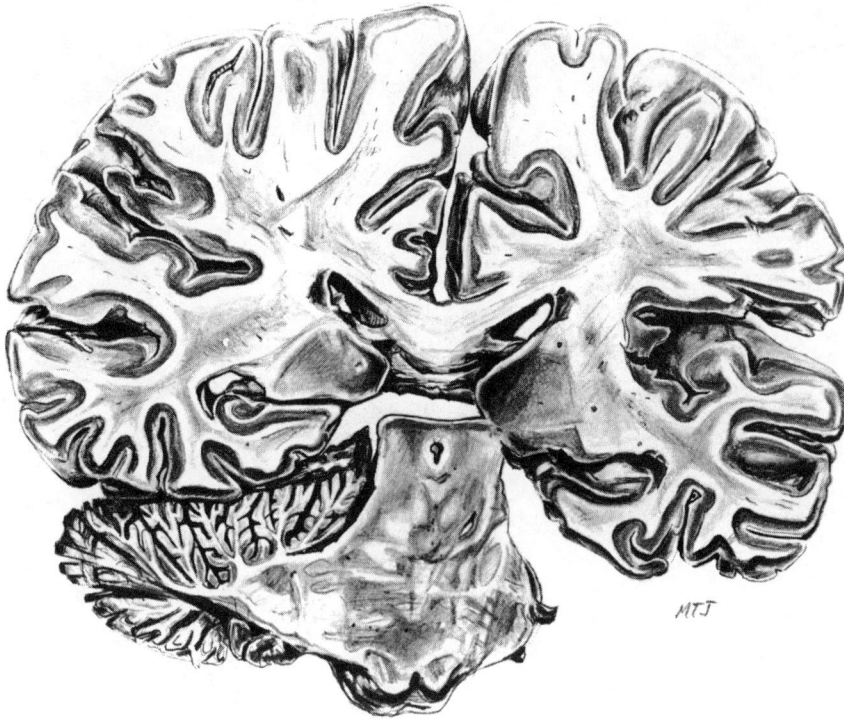

INTRODUCTION

This is a medical procedure to help identify and correct brain chemical imbalance for most types of mental suffering. This method relies partially on medication reactions to guide treatment, but primarily on a concept: That **almost any symptom can be caused by any chemistry** (see graphs in chapter 4). There are basically ten medical treatment categories for the brain, hiding behind approximately 350 clinical diagnoses. These can be moved to the foreground and superimposed over the current system. The method's framework is an aggressive approach which tests, if necessary, most systems of the brain so that the disturbed system(s) can be identified and corrected.

I find this system easier and more effective. For example, **consider the volatile patient.** It is hard clinically to differentiate if they need Prozac, Lithium, Tegretal, Mellaril, Ritalin, Inderal, thyroid or estrogen (females) - see page 56. Unfortunately the reality is the clinical picture can be limited in usefulness. Signs can be too vague to justify any one of these medications. A quick sequential trial of the medications can give clues as to which system is disturbed. Structure to this approach is provided by the protocols, each containing multiple medications, to be tried serially one at a time. Physician energy is saved from the heartache of trying to define something clinically difficult or impossible to differentiate.

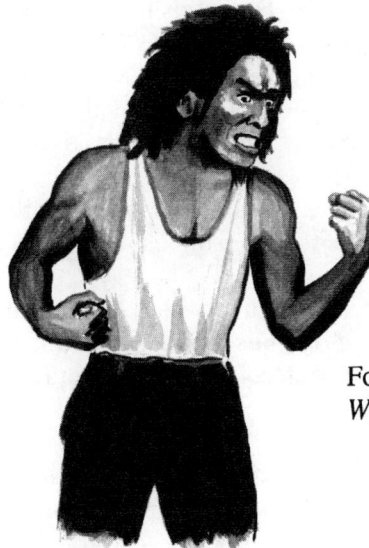

For Temper
Which medicine will work?
Prozac?
Lithium?
Tegretal?
Mellaril?

Furthermore, **medication reactions can be helpful diagnostically** since they reflect underlying brain chemistry (see graph on page 64). Another feature of this system is that **antidotes** are provided for every protocol medication, in case it is needed. I design protocols according to the questions I want answered provided all 9-10 medical catagories are tried quickly if positive results are lacking.

This approach yields surprises; an anorexic teenager with no bipolar symptoms cleared in three hours with lithium. A disabled, panicked, suicidal woman with no symptoms of ADHD cleared in one hour on Ritalin. These observations led me to search for clues to help guide treatment. The answer found was in statistics I compiled and in medication reactions. At times, this was so prominent that I put aside clinical symptoms and let the reactions guide me, until the patients received the medication that would normalize them.

The method is a rapid fire technique where usually **three medications are picked at a time and tried sequentially** to be used as pharmacologic probes to gain understanding of underlying chemistry. Depending on patient reliability and your judgement as a physician, each of the following protocols can be done with one or more visits. Sometimes after brain normalization is achieved, I see that the diagnostic clinical signs and history were actually present, but were too vague to justify the DSM-4 diagnosis. I then appreciate that the medication reactions were prompting reminders, like cue cards, to aid me in not missing the proper diagnosis. **Other times, clues were not present, and the protocol sequences found the defect.** After the problem was identified, fine tuning was done.

In practice, I sometimes blend standard proven treatment with this approach (protocol sequences), which **resembles allergy skin testing.** The hybrid is flexible; if the standard methods are failing, the protocols guide treatment. If the protocols are failing, I return to the standard system. Protocol sequences is a concept I **use to add structure and thoroughness.**

An intriguing concept is that the **protocols, medication reactions and statistics can guide treatment**. A vague or confusing clinical presentation is what this method solves. Patients who clincially look the same can be differentiated using this method. The method decreases the factor of human error. Even if the cause of the imbalance is never identified, correction of the defect is often successful. **This is a finite system for treating an infinite variety of disturbances.** Drug challenge approaches have been increasingly used to assess neurotransmitter function. Provocative testing can either resolve the problem, or reveal more about the underlying chemistry. The protocol method is a rudimentary tool which other doctors can participate in developing further by empirical observation.

Emotionally painful, but hidden chemistry can now be swiftly neutralized. These silent killers may no longer be able to destroy generations of families.

This approach has also been effective in normalizing mental problems due to head injury. **This method should not be used in cases of obvious psychosis** (antidepressants and other medicines could worsen these patients). Yet one woman with constant hallucinations normalized in 30 minutes with Ritalin, and continues to do well with that.

Sometimes having to try many medications can make the patient feel temporarily like a "guinea pig." Yet this approach is comparable to trying on many pairs of shoes before purchase to obtain the best possible fit. If a person is stable enough, I prescribe at each office visit, between 2 and 4 medications (with anti-dotes) so quick comparisons can be made. The search for the "miracle molecule" practically always yields beautiful results, often the same day it is found.

Many patients rush results by compressing each medication trial into 2 or 3 days, though I recommend if possible 5 days per medication. I believe a medicine that takes 6 weeks to work is not as good as one that works in one day.

Limiting medication trials to 5 days or less identifies superior medication matches, and helps to eliminate inferior matches that take longer to work, if they work at all. The standard in the medical field is to pick one antidepressant for six weeks. Yet experience tells me it is more advantageous to quickly compare several medicines to find a favorite.

Patients enthusiastically endorse a **straight forward medical nomenclature.** Frightening labels (for example manic depression or psychotic features) scare patients away. I therefore use words that are less mysterious and more "user friendly." The following labels are based upon **medication actions**, and are a simplification of complex research. (See explanations & references for each on Page 190).

TREATMENT FOR TEN SYSTEMS EFFECTING THE BRAIN

BRAIN CHEMICAL IMBALANCE
Martin T. Jensen, M.D.
Adult & Child Psychiatry

Antidepressants are

1. **Serotonin** and/or
2. **Norepinephrine enhancers.** I call them S and/or NE **agents.**

*Manic depression medications are **"mood stabilizers,"** specifically for unstable NE or unstable electricity.*

3. Lithium is **a "chemical stabilizer."**

4. Depakote and Tegretol are **"electricity smoothers"** or **"stabilizers."**

5. Antipsychotics are **"dopamine reducers"** for elevated dopamine.

6. Stimulants (amphetamines) are **"chemical replacement"** (DA/NE) to correct low blood flow.

7. Anxietolytics (benzodiazepines) **enhance GABA** functioning.

8. Beta adrenergic blockers can **block adrenaline.**

9. **"Thyroid augmentation"** improves metabolic rate.

10. **Estrogen augmentation** may help female estrogen deficiency.

A patient may not like being told they have "psychotic features" if a 4% dose of Stelazine fixes their panic disorder. It is more fair and kinder to say they had a "4% dopamine elevation fixable in one hour." I sense that many doctors, as well as the general population, believe manic depression, psychotic features, and ADHD diagnoses belong to lower functioning individuals. Yet executives, lawyers, politicians, doctors, musicians, performers, etc. frequently have some of this easily correctable chemistry interfering with their lives. Sometimes I discuss medications with the patient in terms of "using access points number 3 or 5" for example, to further destigmatize treatment. This conveys the project is finite and has an end point.

Not enough is known to diagnose a neurochemical defect on the basis of medication response alone. But as a public service, I have tried my best to accurately and approximately describe medication action in simplified terms of brain chemistry.

I feel it is time for physicians to attempt to talk directly about symptoms in physiologic terms. Even if these new chemical labels are not precisely correct yet, the leap can be made. Over time, research will accurately bridge symptoms and chemistry.

METHOD OVERVIEW

In the past when medication choices were few, a 6 week trial period was important. Now that many safe, new medications are available, it is usually possible to find a match that succeeds within 24 hours. The variety of chemical imbalances is infinite. Checking most of the brain's 10 systems is important if results are lacking. Scan systems #1-7 (8 if palpitations are present) for a medicine that helps and does not aggrevate other problem brain circuits. If a bad reaction occurs, the next medication can be started in 1-2 days. If a medicine works 100%, exploration can stop. Instructions for each protocol are written out for the patient. Patients take notes on results. If results in a protocol are mostly poor or adverse, advance to the next protocol. If results are less than 100%, two (and perhaps 3) best medicines (from different systems #1-8), that helped even briefly, are combined, in the lowest effective doses. **This method is not for obvious psychosis.**

PROTOCOL I: Antidepressants 2-4 (but rarely 6) choices tried sequentially and briefly (1 to 7 days each)

	MEDICINE	SYSTEM	PEAK	HALF LIFE
1.	Zoloft		6 hrs.	26 hrs.
	Paxil	low serotonin	5 hrs.	24 hrs.
	Prozac*		7 hrs.	9 days
	Effexor		1.5 hrs.	8 hrs.
	Tofranil	low S/NE	1.5 hrs.	25 hrs.
	Pamelar		—	32 hrs.
2.	Norpramine	low norepinephrine	—	22 hrs.
	Wellbutrin	low DA/NE	2 hrs.	14 hrs.

Antidotes:
(A) Stelazine 2 mg
(B) Xanax 0.25-0.5 mg

* Leave for last due to long half life

PROTOCOL II: Mood Stabilizers, 2-3 tried sequentially, 1-5 days each.
Dopamine Reducer 1 to 3 days

	MEDICINE	SYSTEM	PEAK	HALF LIFE
3.	Eskalith	unstable chemistry	1/2-2 hrs.	22 hrs.
4.	Depakote	unstable electricity	3-4 hrs.	11 hrs.
	Tegretal		4-5 hrs.	15 hrs.
5.	Stelazine	high dopamine	2-4hrs.	—

Antidotes:
(A) Stelazine 2 mg
(B) Xanax 0.25-0.5 mg

——Artane or Xanax

PROTOCOL III: Attention Deficit Disorders (A.D.D.), 3 (rarely 5) tried sequentially, 1-5 days each.

	MEDICINE	SYSTEM	PEAK	HALF LIFE
6.	Tenuate	failure	—	6 hrs.
	Ionamin	(replacement)	—	14 hrs.
	Cylert		3 hrs.	12 hrs
	Ritalin		1.9 hrs.	3 hrs.
	Dexedrine		2 hrs.	10 hrs.

Antidotes:
(A)Stelazine 2 mg
(B) Xanax 0.5 mg

PROTOCOL IV: Anxiety Reducers (for panic patients use from treatment onset as needed until alternative found). 1-3 choices, 1-4 days each.

	MEDICINE	SYSTEM	PEAK	HALF LIFE
7.	Xanax	GABA	1-2 hrs.	11 hrs.
	Ativan	malfunction	2 hrs.	14 hrs.
	Klonopin		1-4 hrs.	23 hrs.

8.	If palpatations are present: Beta adrenergic blocker

PROTOCOL V: Hormonal intervention is considered. **9. Thyroid   10. Estrogen (females)**
See Troubleshooting list on page 49.

PROTOCOL SEQUENCES - BRAIN ASSESSMENT TECHNIQUE

For general mental disorders, **I use this approach unless diagnostic certainty is exceptional i.e.**

Obvious Psychosis or Manic Depression.

Medications that historically failed are not repeated in the protocols unless they were generic. Brand names are used initially as the generics sometimes don't work. **Based on ten medication approaches for the brain, each protocol can be designed to have the two to four medicines most likely to work.** A goal is to try all access points, if necessary, within several visits, to *identify which system is in trouble.* A weakness of standard psychiatry is to use primarily three access points (Serotonin and NE antidepressants, GABA enhancers) rather than ten.

My observations indicate **usually a good match is experienced as such within 24 hours.** Perhaps this is because a precise match on the proper access point works faster than a mismatch. Yet, psychiatric research has proven medications need a longer time to work, for example 3-6 weeks. This may have been true in the past when there were fewer medication choices. Now that a wide variety of safe new medications are available, it is usually possible to find a match that succeeds the same day it is started. Valuable clues can be gathered with 3-5 day trials. Steady-state plasma concentrations are 90% achieved within 4 half-lives of a drug. The graphs in Chapter 5 list half-life data on psychotropic medicines. Backtracking by restarting a medicine for a longer trial may be necessary, yet this is rare. This possible drawback is outweighed by a wealth of objective data (see "Chemical Imbalance Footprints" on page 64) and treatment success that occurs from fluid aggressive trial and error, using carefully designed protocols. Writing instructions for the patient makes multiple medications per protocol more feasible (see page 39).

It is logical to choose the order of the medications in a protocol sequence according to their half-lives, and the drug interactions: If possible, leave the medicine with the longest half-life for last (third) to minimize overlap (for example: Prozac in protocol #1). If necessary, give instructions to wait "x" number of days between medications. I usually recommend **one drug free day between each medication trial.** Xanax or similar medications can be continued for comfort. MAOI's are not being used in the protocols. As fine-tuning is done later, the pace simplifies to titration.

Protocol projects can be tailored according to the patient and the data which needs to be collected. If a patient has already tried multiple medications, protocols can be designed that fill treatment gaps and advance into other protocols. A medication work sheet (see page 37) is useful to overview the brain, organize thoughts and compile medication reactions. Complex medication stories are simplified with this flow sheet. A physical examination should have been done within a year, or sooner, as the situation warrants. Laboratory tests, especially a thyroid test (Free T_4, FTI and TSH) are ordered if necessary.

Follow up visits are usually in 2 weeks for each protocol. Suicidality or other hazards are indications for more frequent visits or hospitalization.

The Following pages contain:
- **Intake Sheet** with accompanying narrative.
- **Worksheet**
- Description of Medication Destabilizations
- An example of a protocol (handwritten for each patient during a visit).
- **Five protocols**

DATE————————————

NAME: ———————————————————————— ( )PHONE ( )——————————

ID. REF.

CC.
Hx.

Sleep:
Ap: Meds Now-
Wt
Temp Intol.
Energy   Hosp:
Hair Loss   Subst-
Brittle Nails
Dry Skin   Suic:
Thyroid FH_x

PAST MEDICAL-   Coffee, Smoke-

Illn-   Surg-

Fam-
                                                       Allerg.
Acci-   Pg/BC/Periods-

FAMILY Hx: Suicidal, Addicted, Temper,
  SOCIAL   Creative, High Energy, Perfection,   Sibs:

               (Personality)   (Work)

F: ( )   —
   m
M:( )   —

_____( )m.   —   Kids:

DEV-Hyper?
Ed-   Occup-   Plans-

Rel/Cul-   Hobbies-   Legal-

Ms:
-Gen Descr.   Mood-   Conc._____Prodctvty_____
-Percep Dist (paranoia, depers., halluc.)_____
-Orientn( ), Memory (rem rec immed)-   Personality_____
-Imp Cont::   Suicide-
               Homicide-
-Judgement
          FUR DIAG ST: PE
                                          Lab-

DX: 1.   TX:

    2.

    3.

34

NARRATIVE OF INTAKE SHEET

ID. Ref. Any identifying or referral information is listed here. City is listed below the phone number.

CC./Hx - Chief complaint and a history of the primary problem.

A **Sleep** description (onset, duration, quality) is obtained.

AP/Wt/Temp Intol/energy/Thyroid FHx:

> **Appetite**, **weight** (including gaining versus losing), and other thyroid symptoms (temperature intolerance, feeling hot or cold much of the time, energy level, hair loss, brittle nails, dry skin, family history of thyroid malfunction) are reviewed.

Hosp. Hospitalizations.

Suic. Suicide attempts and ideas.

Meds now - Current medications are listed with their dosages. A medication reactions history is compiled on the medication work sheet (page 37).

Subst. Substance abuse history. **Coffee** and **smoking** patterns follow.

The **Past Medical** history includes illnesses, medical conditions,

> **Fam**-medical problems that run in the family, **Acci** - accidents, especially with loss of consciousness, **surg** - surgeries,
>
> **Aller** - allergies, **Pg/BC/Periods** - pregnancy, birth control and current menstrual history.

Family Hx (history) and **Social** (history) includes a review of whether anyone in the family or family background had **suicide** problems, breakdowns, alcoholism or **addiction**, **temper** problems, **creativity** (musicians, artists, poets, writers), high **energy** or hyperactivity, or **perfectionistic** traits. **F:( )**, **M:( )** is a description of the father and mother, their ages, **m** if they are married, whether they are alive (what they died of), and what their personalities and dispositions were like, as well as their employment.

> **Siblings** are listed with their emotional problems and employment. _____ **( ) m.** - spouse name, age, marriage duration, personality description and employment are listed here. **Kids** - children are listed with their ages.

Dev-Hyper? - Developmental information about birth, personality and hyperactivity during childhood is addressed. **Ed** - education, **Rel/Cul.** religious or cultural issues are listed here.

Occup - occupation. **Hobbies**, talents, interests are listed - **Plans** - concerning the future. **Legal** - are any legal matters or lawsuits in progress?

MS - Mental status exam with a **gen**eral **descri**ption, **mood**s, **conc**entration, speech **productivity** (markedly increased?), **percep**tual **dist**urbances include paranoia, **depers**onalization, or **halluc**inations (auditory, visual, smells). **Orient**ation and **memory** functioning can be checked (remote, recent and immediate events).

A brief summary of personality traits are listed. Entries for **imp**ulse **cont**rol and **judgement** are also present.

Further diagnostic studies include when last physical exam (**PE**) and laboratory testing (**lab**) were done.

DX - Diagnosis (probable DSM4 axis 1-3).

TX - Treatment ideas including the design of a first protocol of usually 3 medication choices with antidotes. Additional physical exam or laboratory workup needed is recorded.

MEDICATIONS TO REVIEW WITH PATIENT DURING INTAKE

ANTIDEPRESSANTS

Sertraline	ZOLOFT
Paroxetine	PAXIL
Venlafaxine	EFFEXOR
Fluvoxamine	LUVOX
Fluoxetine	PROZAC
Nefazodone	SERZONE
Trazadone	DESYREL
Clomipramine	ANAFRANIL
Amitriptyline	ELAVIL/ENDEP
Perphenazine/Amitriptyline	
	TRIAVIL, ETRAPHON
Doxepin	SINEQUAN/ADAPIN
Trimipramine	SURMONTIL
Imipramine	TOFRANIL
Nortiptyline	PAMELAR
Protriptyline	VIVACTIL
Amoxapin	ASCENDIN
Maprotiline	LUDIOMIL
Desipramine	NORPRAMINE
Bupropian	WELLBUTRIN

Monamine Oxidase Inhibitors

Phenelzine	NARDIL
Tranylcypromine	PARNATE

ANTIPSYCHOTICS

Risperidone	RISPERDAL
Haloperidol	HALDOL
Fluphenazine	PROLIXIN
Thiothixene	NAVANE
Trifluoperazine	STELAZINE
Perphenazine	TRILAFON
Pimozide	ORAP
Molindone	MOBAM
Loxapine	LOXITANE
Chlorprothixene	TARACTIN
Mesoridazine	SERENTIL
Chlorpromazine	THORAZINE
Thioridazine	MELLARIL
Clozapine	CLOZARIL

MOOD STABILIZERS

Lithium	
	ESKALITH CR
	ESKALITH
	LITHOBID
	LITHONATE
	LITHOTABS
	LITHIUM CARBONATE
Lithium Citrate/Liquid	
	LITHIUM CITRATE
Divalproex	DEPAKOTE
Carbamazepine	TEGRETAL

ATTENTION DEFICIT DISORDER TREATMENTS

Methylphenidate	RITALIN TABLET S.R.
Dextroamphetamine	DEXEDRINE TABLET SP.
	DEXTROSTAT
Phentermine	IONAMINE
Diethylpropion	TENUATE
Pemoline	CYLERT
Clonidine	CATAPRES

LONG ACTING ANTIPSYCHOTICS

Haloperidol Decanoate	
	HALDOL DECANOATE
Fluphenazine Decanoate	
	PROLIXIN DECANOATE
Fluphenazine Enanthate	
	PROLIXIN ENANTHATE

SIDE EFFECT MEDICINES

Biperiden	AKINETON
Trihexyphenidyl	ARTANE
Diphenhydramine	BENADRYL
Benztropine	COGNETIN
Procyclidine	KEMADRIN
Amantadine	SYMMETREL
Dantrolen	DANTRIUM
Bromocriptine	PARLODEL

ANXIETY REDUCER MEDICINES

Alprazolam	XANAX
Chlordiazepoxide	LIBRIUM
Clonazepam	KLONOPIN
Clorazepate	TRANZENE
Diazepam	VALIUM
Lorazepam	ANTIVAN
Oxazepam	SERAX
Buspirone	BUSPAR
Propranolol	INDERAL

Sleepers

Estazolam	PROSOM
Flurazepam	DALMANE
Quazepam	DORAL
Temazepam	RESTORIL
Triazolam	HALCION
Zolpidem	AMBIEN
Chloral Hydrate	
Hydroxyzine	VISTARIL

THYROID

T_3 Lieothyronine	CYTOMEL
T_4 Levothyroxine	LEVOTHROID
Levothyroxine	LEVOXYL
Levothyroxine	SYNTHROID
Mixture	ARMOUR
Mixture	SPT
Mixture	THYRAR
Mixture	THYROLAR

Name:_____

WORKSHEET FOR BRAIN SYSTEMS - Compile Reactions

I   Antidepressants

1. Serotonin
       Zoloft
       Paxil
       Serzone
       Luvox
       Prozac

   Mixed (S/N)
       Effexor
       Tofranil
       Pamelar
       MAOI - Nardil/Parnate
2. Norepinephrine
       Norpramine
   DA/NE
       Wellbutrin

II   Mood Stabilizers (NE or Electrical Instability)

3.   Lithium

4.   Depakote
         Tegretal

5. **Dopamine Elevation**

         Stelazine
         Mellaril
         Risperdal
         Haldol

III   6. Attention Deficit Disorders (DA/NE failure)

         Cylert
         Tenuate
         Ritalin
         Ionamin
         Dexedrine

IV   7. GABA
         Xanax
         Ativan
         Klonopin
         Valium

8. **Adrenaline Blockers**
         Inderal/Tenormin

V   9. Thyroid
         Cytomel
         Synthroid

10. **Estrogen** (females)

DESCRIPTIONS OF MEDICATION DESTABILIZATIONS

As destabilization occurs on a medication, the graphs in the next chapter can provide statistics for medication choices.

ANTIDEPRESSANT DESTABILIZATION

Emotional Destabilization triggered by antidepressants include any of the following: Patients may feel worse, more anxious, confused, labile, distressed, dazed, "in a fog", fatigued, exhausted, weak, shaky, "hyper", agitated, violent, suicidal, scattered with thinking, dulled, "zombied", like crying, bizarrely elated, wired", or "amped". Also the medication may have worked then stopped working despite increasing dosage. They can have nightmares or hallucinations. Presenting complaints may intensify. One antidepressant may cause problems while another does not.

Somatic (Physical) Destabilization triggered by antidepressants may include any of the following: rapid heart rate, palpitations, diarrhea, headaches, sweating, restless legs, flushing, speech impairment, or increased craving for whatever addiction was their problem (food, alcohol, drugs, etc.). Weight gain with a weight loss type of antidepressant can also be an example of this. Extreme levels of physical side-effects (nausea, headaches, etc.) raises suspicion that physical destabilization is occurring. Sedation by an activating antidepressant is also usually destabilization.

LITHIUM DESTABILIZATION

Mental Worsening can occur from a low dose of lithium. This can be characterized by **distress, agitation, confusion, loss of coordination, sedation,** or an accentuation of normal side effects. This usually means lithium is the wrong medication.

DEPAKOTE DESTABILIZATION

Patients may feel worse, moody, tense, agitated, get a headache, or become very sedated at a normal dose. The medication may initially work, then stop working. Sometimes these are just side effects, but more often signify a different underlying chemistry is present.

TEGRETAL DESTABILIZATION

Patients may feel worse, uneasy, agitated, stressed, fidgety, confused, volatile, weak, "zombied", like their skin is "crawling", sweaty or uncoordinated at a normal dose. This can destabilize like an antidepressant. The medication may initially work, then stop working. Sometimes these are just side effects, but more often signify a different underlying chemistry is present.

ANTIPSYCHOTIC DESTABILIZATION

A patient taking antipsychotic may feel worse, confused, agitated, irritable, "wired", or have nightmares. Often these are just side effects (Akathisia - page 144). Yet sometimes these symptoms signify that there is no dopamine elevation, and that a different underlying chemistry is present.

STIMULANT DESTABILIZATION

A patient taking stimulant may feel worse, moody, irritable, volatile, confused, agitated, destructive, sad, or "speedy". Palpitations, hallucinations or severe insomnia can occur. If the medicine initially worked neuroleptic may need to be added, or the stimulant may need to be switched to a different one. The above destabilization signs can be side effects or signify that a different underlying chemistry is present.

BENZODIAZEPINE DESTABILIZATION

Sometimes patients taking this can feel much worse, depressed, labile, moody, agitated or distressed. One variety of benzodiazepine might cause this while others do not. This may be a side effect, but usually reflects different underlying chemistry is present.

THYROID DESTABILIZATION

A patient taking thyroid may feel worse, agitated, anxious, confused, insomnic, disorganized, disoriented, or hyperactive. They may be taking excessive thyroid, or have a different underlying chemical imbalance.

*Example of instructions to patient with panic disorder
given during first visit*

1. Stop prior medicine – let it clear from body for 1–2 days.
2. <u>Zoloft 50 mg</u>: 1/2–1 tablet in a.m. for 3–5 days.

   Antidote – if worse, stop the medicine

   – "going nuts" – Stelazine 2 mg

   – "anxious" – Xanax 0.25 mg

3. Stop Zoloft, let it clear for a day,

   start <u>Paxil 20 mg</u>: 1/2–1 tablet in a.m. for 3–5 days.

   Antidote – same as above.

4. Stop Paxil, let it clear for a day,

   start <u>Prozac 20 mg</u>:   1 in a.m. for 3–5 days.

   Antidote – same as above.

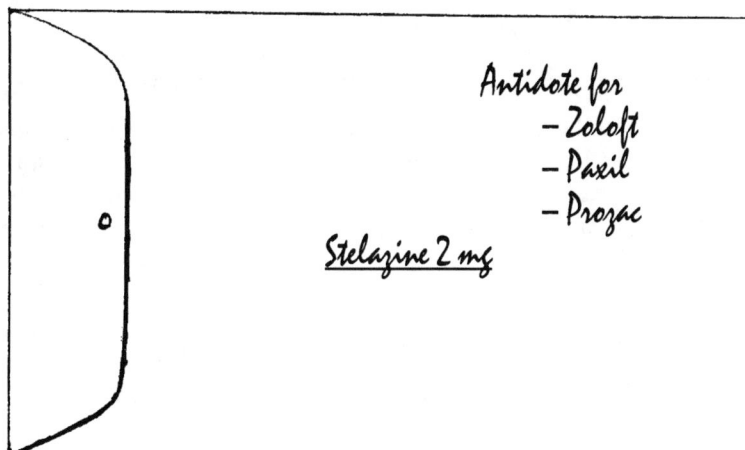

Antidote for
– Zoloft
– Paxil
– Prozac

<u>Stelazine 2 mg</u>

PROTOCOLS 1-5

Protocol #1: Antidepressants (2-4) per visit. (SE, NE enhancement)

Try each medication one at a time for 3 to 5 days, but discontinue it sooner if an adverse reaction occurs. Until more is understood, it is important to compare briefly an assortment of antidepressants. I am amazed to watch how each person usually prefers one strongly over all others, and that the best results occur typically within a day. In my opinion, limiting medication trial to five days or less helps to identify superior matches and eliminate inferior ones; an antidepressant may have parts that can be misread by the brain and body to cause adverse reactions.

Can an antidepressant be found that fits and does not aggravate underlying problem circuits?

Serotonin Enhancers

A. **Zoloft** 50mg (#7) daily in a.m., 3-5 days, then
B. **Paxil** 20mg (#7) daily in a.m., 3-5 days, then
C. **Prozac** 20mg (#7) daily in a.m., 3-5 days,
D. Serzone 150mg (#7) ½-1 twice daily for 3 days, then
E. Luvox 50mg (#7) 1 in a.m., 3-5 days.

I might typically prescribe F, A, B, J and C in two visits to be tried one at a time, 3-5 days each, with a "washout" day between medications. Note that long-acting Prozac is tried last so minimal overlap will occur in the sequence. The patients record results on a reaction data sheet.

While traditional tricylics (G, H, I) are sometimes best, they are less safe in overdose and may have more side effects. The safest antidepressants may be chosen before other antidepressants as a first approach (A, B, C, D, E, F, J). Pharmaceutical companies can supply doctors with samples for protocol 1. Antidotes (from my office) are supplied in a small envelope with the samples:

> Antidote: Stelazine 2mg - #3, or Xanax 0.5 mg - #3

They can be taken if severe emotional destabilization occurs. Relief comes in 1-2 minutes if the broken tablet is held in the mouth briefly (30 seconds) before being washed down, while simply swallowing the pill is calming in 2-15 minutes and rarely takes an hour. After a negative reaction has been neutralized, the patient can try the next medication in 1-2 days. It is considerate and safer with protocols to provide an emergency antidote for every medication "probe."

Xanax 0.25-0.5 mg is supplied from the start for panic disorder patients, but they are encouraged to try antidepressants alone and use the Xanax only if needed. It is also helpful if the stelazine antidote fails (rare). The above group of medicine samples with antidotes are loaded into a small bag, and instructions are written.

If a medication was clearly successful, it is prescribed for a one-month trial (adjusted, refilled as needed) and further exploration is stopped.

NE stimulating antidepressant choices include the following:

> F. **Effexor** 37.5 mg (#10) - 1 at breakfast and 2 p.m. daily, then
> G. Tofranil 25 mg (#15) - 1-3 at bedtime daily, then
> H. Pamelar 10 mg (#15) - 1-3 at bedtime daily, then
> I. Norpramin 10 mg (#15) - 1-5 in a.m. daily, then
> J. **Wellbutrin** 75 mg (#10) - 1 at breakfast and 2 p.m. daily.

If these are tried before protocol 2 and 3, **recognize that as each medicine fails, it becomes more urgent to advance to protocol 2.**

The principal of my method is to limit protocol #1 (antidepressants) to 3, and perhaps 4 "best choices" which are briefly compared. The result is the patient either improves, or the diagnostic evaluation switches to other brain systems which are then quickly explored (protocols 2-5). **Protocol 1 is perhaps a crude litmus test for "reactive," unstable, toxic or failing brain chemistry** (protocols 2-5).

Worsening or poor results by multiple antidepressants historically or in protocol #1 justify advancing to protocol 2. **This boundary may be the strongest factor leading to successful treatment.** The adverse reactions medically suggest some type of reactivity is in the brain that should be neutralized by protocols 2-5.

If an antidepressant caused worsening, the following is a summary of which medicine(s) finally gave a lasting excellent result for 275 of my patients in 1995:

> — another antidepressant 30%
> — chemical or electrical stabilization 15%
> — dopamine reduction 11%
> — chemical replacement 20%
> — GABA enhancement 18%
> — thyroid enhancement 6%

If an **antidepressant initially worked well, but then caused worsening** (in hours, days or months), this can often be gently corrected. To normalize a contaminating problematic circuit, try adding one of the following to the antidepressant (or switch to another more compatible antidepressant):

> Light Destabilization Controllers for Antidepressants:
>
> a. Stelazine 2 mg or Risperdal 1 mg each morning *or*
> b. Depakote 250 mg each morning *or*
> c. Eskalith 300 mg each morning

Hopefully, an antidepressant may be found that will not aggravate other problem circuits. If these unstable chemistries are too major a factor, they must be moved to the foreground and neutralized directly (protocols 2-5).

PROTOCOL #2: Mood (chemical and electrical) Stabilizers (3), Dopamine Reduction

If no results occurred or bad reactions happened in Protocol #1, advance to the mood stabilizers. This is for patients who usually react adversely to antidepressants. Medication trials can be brief to gain clues. Patients appreciate having medical proof (protocol 1 failure) that mood stabilizer trials are indicated. They are able to rate each; i.e. "chemical stabilization helped 100%, and electricity smoothing helped 25%." Since doses are low and brief, toxicity in this phase is not too relevant. Of course healthy kidneys and liver are important for lithium and Depakote respectively.

For up to 5 days each:

A. Eskalith 300mg (#15) one in A.M., perhaps one at
  noon, perhaps one at dinner
  then:
B. Depakote 250mg (#15) 1/2-1 three times daily,
  then: (especially if anxious)
  Tegretal 100mg (#15) two or three times daily
  (especially if frustrated)

 Medications should be discontinued if adverse reactions occur. An antidote which can provide comfort for this Protocol is:

Antidote: Stelazine 2 mg or Xanax 0.5 mg

Tegretal structurally resembles a tricyclic antidepressant. If worsening occurs from Tegretal, Stelazine 2mg can be a more effective antidote.

If a mood stabilizer works, patients may still like to compare this with other mood stabilizers. Some prefer a single Eskalith CR 450mg tablet each morning.

Many of the medications of protocol 2, 3, and 4 in tablet form can work within 2 minutes if placed for 30-60 seconds within the mouth before being swallowed with water. This can be useful for unpredictable upsetting crises. It also may help a patient who forgot to take medication.

A neuroleptic is tried next to check for dopamine elevation.

C. Stelazine 2mg (#10) - 1 in A.M. daily

Occasionally restless "akathisia" (page 144) can occur even at this low dose. Switching to Risperdal 1 mg twice daily can clarify if a dopamine toxicity was present. The antidote for worsening is Xanax 0.5 mg.

PROTOCOL #3: Attention Deficit (Hyperactivity) Disorder Treatment (Chemical Replacement)

If all has failed, it is time to recognize that what is probably occurring is chemical failure (ADHD chemistry) and/or GABA malfunction. These have the most adverse medication reactions of any psychiatric diagnoses. Because symptoms are vague, chemical failure is the most common cause of treatment failure until it is correctly identified. One of the strongest features of my method is that this obscure and often missed chemistry gets discovered and fixed. Some of the victims appear quite ordinary except for their distress, panic, or depression. Many were never hyperactive. Children are probably being overtreated for ADHD, while adults are being undertreated.

This protocol focuses on the DA/NE system, and its probable failure.

The most successful choices should be tried first for up to 5 days each, one at a time:

> **A. Ritalin** 5mg tabs (#15) - 1 at 8 A.M., noon, 4 P.M. daily,
> then
> **B. Dexedrine** 5mg tabs (#15) - 1/2-1 at 8 A.M., noon,
> 4 P.M. daily, then
> **C. Cylert** 37.5mg chewable (#5) - 1/2-1 at 8 A.M. daily

If an intolerable reaction occurs, the medication is discontinued, and an antidote may be taken:

> Antidote: Stelazine 2mg and/or Xanax 0.5mg

Note that the Ritalin is taken in a dose 1-4% of that which is typical of drug abuse doses, and gently replaces a brain chemical which is mising. Tolerance and addiction should not occur in this setting. For Ritalin, the usual dose range is 5-20mg, 3 times daily. Generic Ritalin is often weaker than brand name.

If results were good, but worsening followed, dopamine reduction typically in a 3-8% range corrects this (**Stelazine** 2mg daily with the stimulant). The percentage is based on the fraction of a full neuroleptic dose which is required. Sometimes **Eskalith** 300mg in the AM prevents worsening (simultaneous chemical failure and chemical instability were present).

> Light Destabilization controllers for DA/NE Rx:
>
> a. Stelazine 2 mg each morning
>   Mellaril 10-30 mg at bedtime if insomnia
>   *or*
> b. Eskalith 300 mg each morning

Other times stimulants initially work, then destabilize into agitation, crying, and confusion, until the medicine is stopped. Perhaps this is where amphetamines got their treacherous reputation.

> Antidote: Stelazine 2 mg and/or Xanax 0.5 mg

Whether Ritalin, Dexedrine or Cylert worked or failed, it is good next to **compare a variety of NE stimulating antidepressants** (see page 41) to see if a less controversial solution can be found. The search for the perfect molecule that works exceptionally, and in hours, is worth this trouble.

> *The spectrum of A.D.D. chemistries appears to be wide. The medicines that work have DA/NE like structure or subunits that the brain can use. If the match is poor, nerve binding without functioning can cause worsening of DA/NE failure and an adverse reaction; the correct ADD medicine (if this is known) is the best antidote.*

Alternatively attempts can first be made to **find a more suitable match** for the failed DA/NE. **Dexadrine** and **Ritalin** are both FDA approved for ADHD. Gentler "diet pills" for chemical replacement may produce a better result. For example, Wellbutrin, then Ritalin destabilized an ADHD patient into crying, irritability, and distress. **Tenuate** 25 mg twice daily gave complete and stable relief. Tenuate is a diet pill resembling the antidepressant Wellbutrin (see page 57).

Both Ionamin and Tenuate are diet pills that are not approved for ADHD by the FDA. Prescribing an approved medication for unapproved use does not violate any law. Physicians are not restricted by indications and labeling of the Food and Drug Administration (FDA). The FDA's failure to describe a medication use may be due to the pharmaceutical company not knowing, and thus not notifying the FDA to review this aspect of a medication's effectiveness. Few doctors realize the treatment latitude they possess, and mistakenly view FDA guidelines as absolute and authoritative.(Reference 3)

Having scientific rationale for treatment can be a guiding principal. For example it is logical that mild ADD, unresponsive to Wellbutrin, can be treated with a mild amphetamine such as Ionamin, which structurally resembles dexedrine, or Tenuate which structurally resembles Wellbutrin. Thus stronger amphetamine (Ritalin or Dexedrine) with their complicated dose schedules may sometimes be avoided. Diet pills don't require triplicate prescriptions and thus are easier to write.

A standard ADHD agent, **Cylert**, has a reputation for being weaker. Yet many adults clearly benefit most from Cylert.

MAOI's such as Nardil and Parnate are more dangerous than stimulants (see page 137), and yet sometimes more reliably control adult ADHD distress. Be aware that **chemical failure often requires a very specific match. One agent may work completely while all others cause decompensation** or require dopamine reduction.

As a physician I am concerned that amphetamine addicts may read this book and try to abuse this method by providing a doctor with false medication reactions in order to obtain stimulant. Hopefully these people could get their imbalance fixed by Protocol #1, or #2. If their chemistry is stable enough, they could take Norpramine to decrease amphetamine craving. Attention deficit disordered amphetamine abusers do exist. Wellbutrin, Cylert, or stimulant, under close medical supervision can be effective.

Two brain chemical imbalances are treated with potentially addictive medications. It has been proven with ADHD (DA/NE lack) that **amphetamine** replacement treatment is not addictive. I believe this also applies with GABA. A poorly functional GABA system (proven by failure of other protocols) may require long term, low dose **benzodiazepine.** It is my observation that tolerance does not result in this situation. Of course in this group, these medications taken in excess, lead to tolerance and addiction. The **opiate** medications supersede and diminish stress from most chemical imbalances. Thus during surgery, psychotropics can often be discontinued if opiate is given. Caution should be exercised however against suddenly lowering GABA agents or thyroid medicine dosages.

There are combinations of chemical imbalance that are more difficult to treat. When chemical failure occurs with chemical instability or low serotonin, the medicines for this (lithium, serotonin enhancers) can worsen ADD or ADHD distress.

PROTOCOL #4: Anxiety: GABA Enhancement
                                     Adrenaline Blockers

- If results are still lacking, GABA deficiency is frequently the cause. GABA **depressions can be as dangerous** as attention deficit disorders and bipolar depressions. A low dose benzodiazepine usually solves this. Just as ADD chemistry can result in **many adverse medication reactions**, so can poor GABA functioning. The most effective benzodiazepine should be selected. Sometimes one works when others failed (see page 74)

- Beta adrenergic blockers block adrenaline and may be helpful in hours when cardiac palpitations and panic are present.

> Inderal 40 mg: 1/2-1 three times daily

For panic disorder patients, medicines from Protocol #4 can be blended with protocol 1, 2 or 3 as needed from the onset of treatment. As the chemical imbalance is solved, it may be possible to taper or stop protocol #4.

The best 2 or even 3 medications from different systems are blended if necessary.

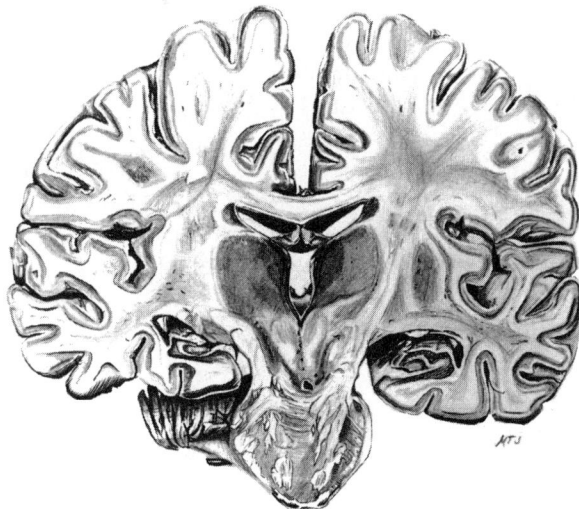

75%-90% of the brain's neurons have GABA

PROTOCOL #5: HORMONAL; THYROID
ESTROGEN (FEMALES)

Thyroid:

A thyroid dysfunction can cause resistant **fatigue** or **weight gain**. Thyroid labs can be normal, but clues are frequently found in the past history, family history, and sometimes other thyroid symptoms such as **temperature intolerance**, **hair loss**, **dry skin** and **brittle nails**. **Adverse reactions to antidepressants** are often present. Giving these patients low dose thyroid usually corrects fatigue, weight gain and other thyroid signs, but not panic or severe depression. Yet occasionally, thyroid medicine alone in a 5-8% dose completely clears all symptoms. The patient in this situation had "thyroid reserves that were 5% depleted."

The thyroid gland determines the speed of all chemical reactions in the body and brain. The surface of the brain (cerebrum) contains probably 100 billion neurons. Over 90% of patients with low thyroid functioning are normal by standard lab tests (Reference 25). Most thyroid "differences" are due to an inherited defect in the immune system, causing autoimmune attack on the thyroid gland.

"Subclinical", borderline, or impending hypothyroidism may progress to overt hypothyroidism. It may, however, continue for years without confirmation from laboratory tests. Occasionally thyroid functioning is excessive rather than deficient. Sometimes patients who are hot and exhausted have other chemical imbalances.

Thyroid dysfunction can simply be a genetic difference as reflected by a positive family history of thyroid disturbance. This can cause or amplify abnormalities in any of the ten medical systems effecting the brain. A mildly hypothyroid woman who could not tolerate antidepressants, could after starting thyroid replacement, yet this seems to be the exception. Most **thyroid-different patients** need one or two of the ten medical approaches to feel well. Sensitive clues of thyroid dysfunction are in the table on the next page.

It is as if a thyroid difference is the "wild card" that can convert normal chemistry to any other chemistry (protocol 1-5). See the graph on page 58, and detailed neurotransmitter data from studies on page 24.

Low thyroid reserve is the single most common biochemical abnormality in psychiatric patients (Reference 23) See page 111-112 and 151 for thyroid lab work.

Thyroid medication, if indicated, usually follows completion of the protocol for other brain systems. Synthroid 25-50mcg. (8-16% dose) daily or Cytomel 5-25mcg. (5-25% dose) daily, are typically helpful. Cytomel has a shorter half-life (1 day), but sometimes too much potency (T_3) and fluctuating levels.

If thyroid hormone causes worsening, antidotes include any of the following:

> a. Stelazine 2mg (bizarreness, volatility)
> b. Eskalith 300mg (crying)
> c. Inderal 40mg (palpitations)
> d. Xanax 0.25-0.5mg (anxiety)

THYROID CHECKLIST
ARE ANY PRESENT?

☐ POSITIVE FAMILY HISTORY

☐ WEIGHT GAIN, OR LOSS: _____LBS.

☐ COLD OR HEAT INTOLERANCE

☐ LETHARGY, LOW ENERGY, FATIGUE

☐ HAIR LOSS ☐ BRITTLE NAILS ☐ DRY SCALY SKIN

☐ DEPRESSION, ANXIETY ☐ ENLARGED NECK BASE

☐ LABS: (Always ordered if any of above signs are present, yet results are only sometimes helpful.)

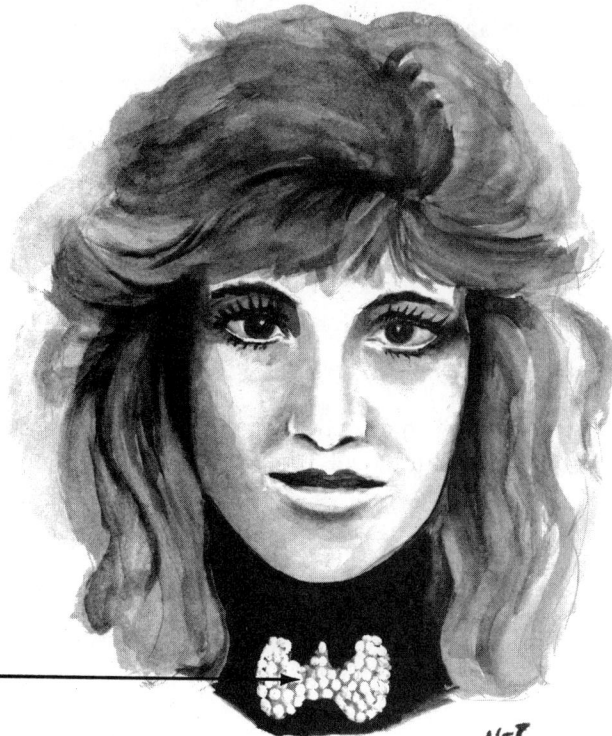

Thyroid Gland ————

47

ESTROGEN

Women can have low estrogen causing emotional problems, panic, or decreased sex drive. Some improve with estrogen stimulation to the brain. Those not low in estrogen may get worse when more is added. There may exist low estrogen levels or the brain may be lacking in responsiveness to estrogen. Lab testing for FSH, LH and estrogen is only erratically helpful in premenopausal females. The clinical picture of **emotional problems is the most helpful index.**

It is important a physical exam be done before estrogen treatment and annually thereafter.

If birth control is needed, an **oral contraceptive** is selected. Some formulations cause adverse reactions, while others help emotionally by providing a consistent estrogen level. Estrogen can cause worsening. For females older than 35-45, oral contraceptives are considered to have more risks than a combination of

> oral Premarin 0.625 mg
> and Progesterone 2.5 mg (if uterus present)

taken on days 1-25 of each month, then stopped to allow withdrawal bleeding. The use of progesterone on days 14-25 of each month appears to eliminate uterine cancer risk (reference 8).

If response is still poor, another approach can be tried:

> Monthly IM shots of Estradiol 10ml - lasts 4 weeks
> and one Estrone 2.5 mg tablet - immediate acting

If a family history of breast cancer is present, this approach should not be used (see page 152).

Menopause is characterized by erratic menses, which stop, hot flashes, night sweats, and decreased vaginal lubrication. FSH and LH increase as estrogen diminishes.

Gynecologists and family practitioners have more experience with this estrogen approach than I have. Very rarely do I get to this level in the protocols.

TROUBLE SHOOTING IF ALL PROTOCOLS FAIL

1. An underlying medical condition could be interfering with results. Refer to the organicity checklists in Chapter 6, page 79.

2. Substance abuse may be contaminating results.

3. Check that medication trials were adequate (dosage,duration), ie. at least 5 days when results were vague or questionable.

4. Consider brief trials of antidepressants that were missed: Serzone/Luvox/ Effexor/Tofranil/Pamelar/Norpramine. If results were initially good, then worse, add a destabilization controller (page 41).

5. Consider Attention Deficit Disorder medications that were missed. If results were initially good, then worse, add a destabilization controller (page 43).

6. Standard psychiatry would recommend a 6 week trial of whichever antidepressant was most promising, yet if #4 failed, I have not seen this work.

7. Occasionally pure, severe GABA malfunction occurs: see protocol 4. Raise the dose of benzodiazepine.

8. Consider an MAOI, as a last choice, for resistant panic or depression (rare).

9. Review standard treatment methods and see if anything was missed (very rare).

Adrenergic effects vs. Anti-Adrenergic effects

Page 172

Antidepressants Stimulants Thyroid	Mood stabilizers (Lithium, Depakote) Antipsychotics (low dose) GABA agents Beta Blockers

If adrenergic medicines are causing worsening, they should be lowered, stopped, or changed. If many adrenergic medicines fail, anti-adrenergics can be used with the best adrenergic, or instead of any adrenergic.

STATISTICS FROM MY PRACTICE

A Variety of Subtypes for Most Mental Disorders Were Identified and Corrected Using a Protocol Sequence of Ten Medical Approaches.

Most neurotransmitter systems connect to each of the brains main structures. A defect in any one transmitter system thus can cause failure of that brain function.

Most behavioral functions depend on all neurotransmitter systems being intact. The result: Any symptom can be caused by a defect in almost any transmitter.

- *Statistics were from the past year of private practice in Southern California.*
- *One medication was tried at a time, except for "GABA comfort" (benzodiazepines) which was available as needed during protocols.*
- *Using the protocol method, SSRI's were used as the antidepressant access point, norepinephrine and other antidepressants were used much less [the serotonin system for the most part, feeds into the norepinephrine system]. Beta adrenergic receptor blockers, and estrogen results were not compiled.*

CONTENTS: GRAPHS

LEGEND

AD - Antidepressant

1.   ▦   Serotonin (SSRI's)

         〰   Mixed (S/NE)

2.   ▨   Norepinphrine (NE)

         ⁖   s, NE, Dopamine (DA)
                 [Wellbutrin]

3. **Li** - Lithium (Chemical Stabilizer)

4. **Elec** - Electricity Stabilizers
            D - Depakote
            T - Tegretal

5. **AP** - Antipsychotic (DA Reduction)

6. **St** - Stimulant (Chemical Replacement)

7. **G** - GABA - Benzodiazepines

8. Beta adrenergic blockers were not recorded in most graphs.

9. **Thyr** - Thyroid Malfunction

         S   - Symptoms or Family History
         B   - Borderline Labs
         +   - Labs Positive For Hypothyroidsm

         Rx   *Thyroid replacement medicine prescribed*

Thyroid usually was a factor, but not a cure,
so was set apart in most graphs

10. Estrogen was not recorded.

PANIC / ANXIETY

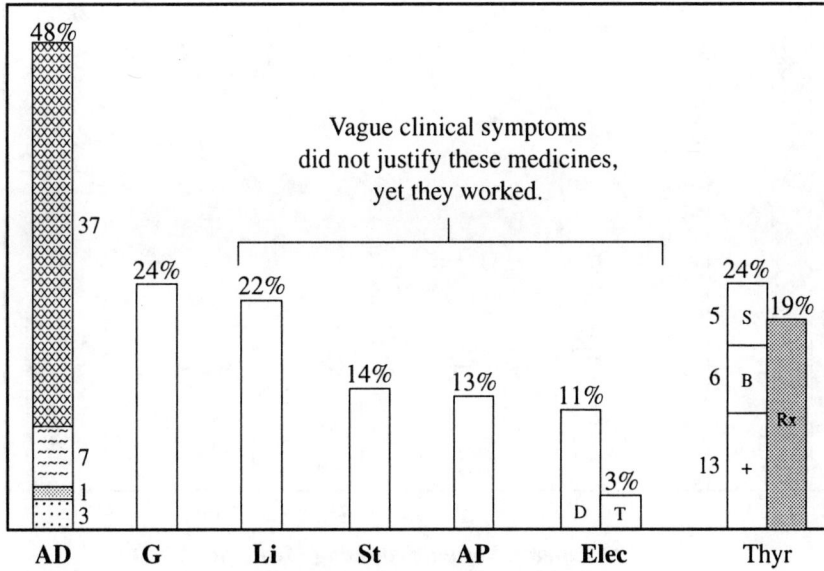

48%

37

Vague clinical symptoms
did not justify these medicines,
yet they worked.

24%

22%

24%

5 | S

19%

14%

13%

6 | B

11%

Rx

7

3%

13 | +

1
3

D | T

AD   **G**   **Li**   **St**   **AP**   **Elec**   Thyr

94 Patients Normalized Using Medicine

Blends in 35%

Stimulant required a low 4-6% antipsychotic dose, 21% of the time (not recorded in graph).

Beta adrenergic blockers such as inderal, were not recorded, yet were sometimes helpful, especially for palpitations.

Estrogen was not recorded, yet was sometimes helpful.

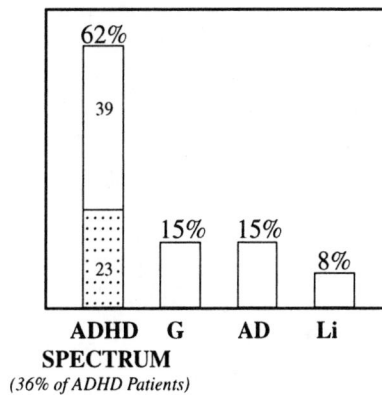

62%

39

15%   15%

8%

23

ADHD   **G**   **AD**   **Li**
SPECTRUM
(36% of ADHD Patients)

Most panic victims got worse with coffee, yet others enjoyed coffee.
What was this chemistry?

13 patients who had panic, but not from coffee.

D E P R E S S I O N

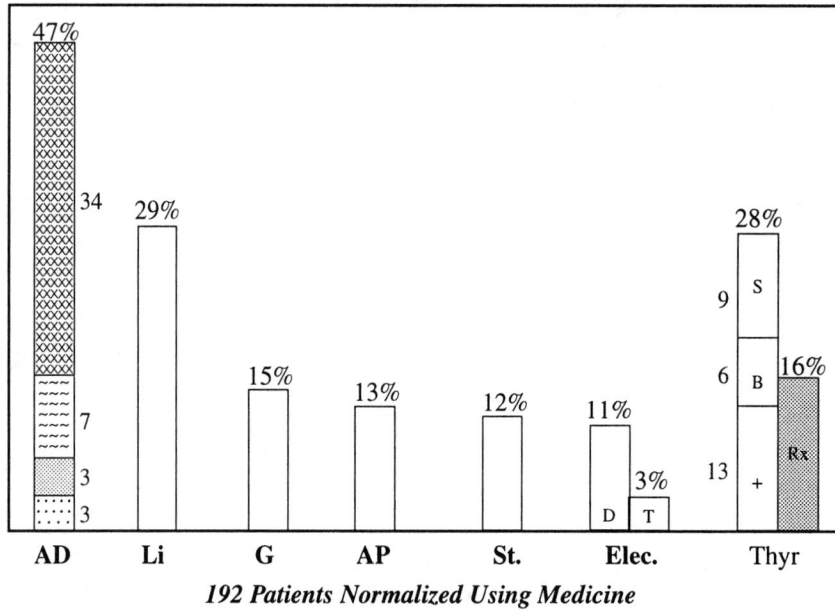

192 Patients Normalized Using Medicine

Blends in 43% (my patient population was very ill).
*

Stimulant required a 4-6% antipsychotic dose, 25% of the time, and was not recorded in the graph.

SUICIDALITY

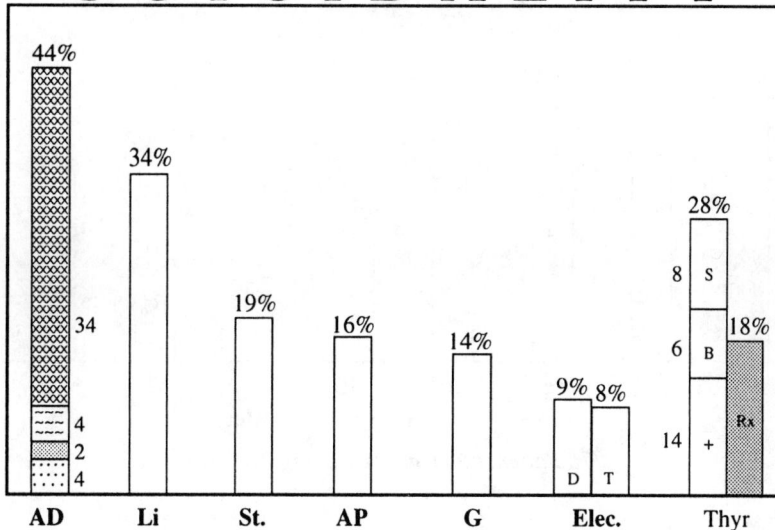

44%

34

4
2
4

34%

19%

16%

14%

28%

8 | S

6 | B

14 | +

18%

Rx

9% 8%

D | T

AD   **Li**   **St.**   **AP**   **G**   **Elec.**   Thyr

134 Suicidal Patients Normalized Using Medicine

Blends in 39%

A majority of patients who attempted suicide, and responded to an SSRI, got well with Zoloft.

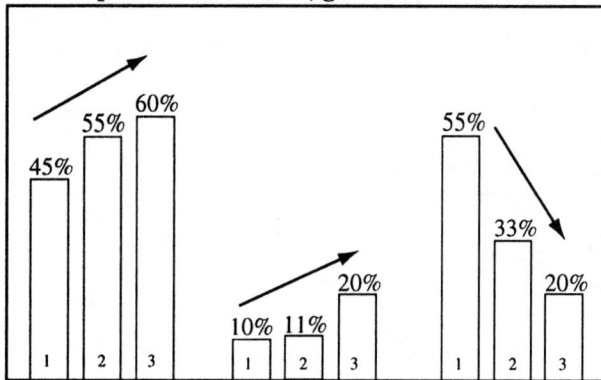

45% 55% 60%

1   2   3

ZOLOFT

10% 11% 20%

1   2   3

PAXIL

46 Patients

55%

33% 20%

1   2   3

PROZAC

3 Levels of Suicidality

1 - **Mild** Suicide Thoughts
2 - **Severe** Suicide Thoughts
3 - **History** of Suicide Attempts

It was important patients compare SSRI's since most had a favorite.

If suicide attempts occurred in the past, note how antidepressants became less helpful, and other medicines more helpful.

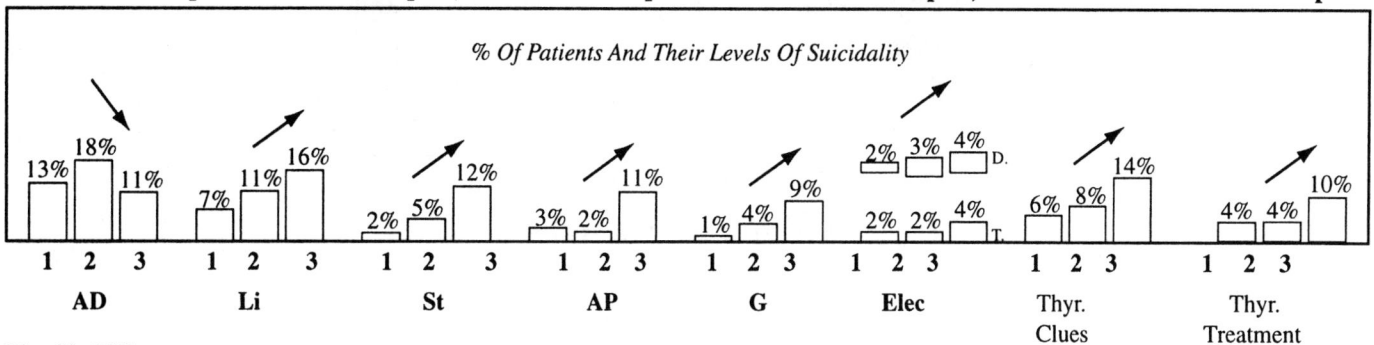

% Of Patients And Their Levels Of Suicidality

| 13% | 18% | 11% | | 7% | 11% | 16% | | 2% | 5% | 12% | | 3% | 2% | 11% | | 1% | 4% | 9% | | 2% | 3% | 4% D. | | 6% | 8% | 14% | | 4% | 4% | 10% |

| 1 | 2 | 3 | | 1 | 2 | 3 | | 1 | 2 | 3 | | 1 | 2 | 3 | | 1 | 2 | 3 | | 1 | 2 | 3 T. | | 1 | 2 | 3 | | 1 | 2 | 3 |

AD   **Li**   **St**   **AP**   **G**   **Elec**   Thyr. Clues   Thyr. Treatment

Blend in 39%

55

TEMPER, IRRITABILITY, HATE, VIOLENCE

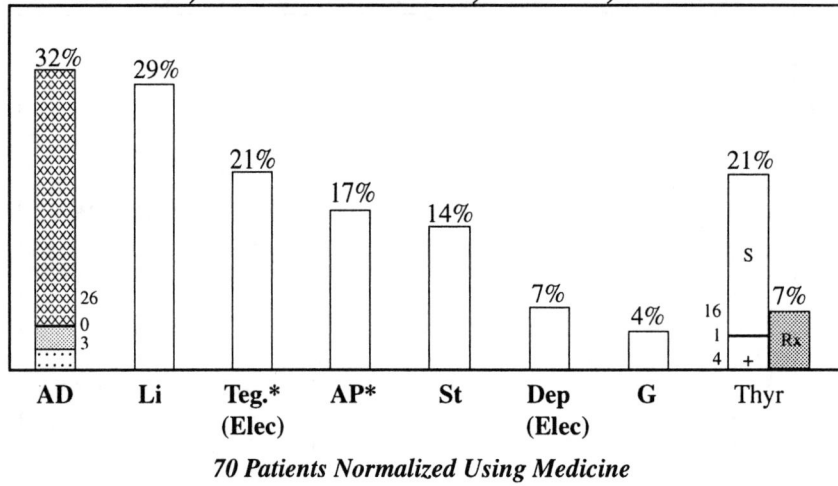

32% 29% 21% 17% 14% 7% 4% 21% 7%

26
0
3

16
1
4

S
+
Rx

AD   Li   Teg.*   AP*   St   Dep   G   Thyr
           (Elec)   (Elec)

70 Patients Normalized Using Medicine

Blends in 31%
*Violence Prominent

BIZARRENESS

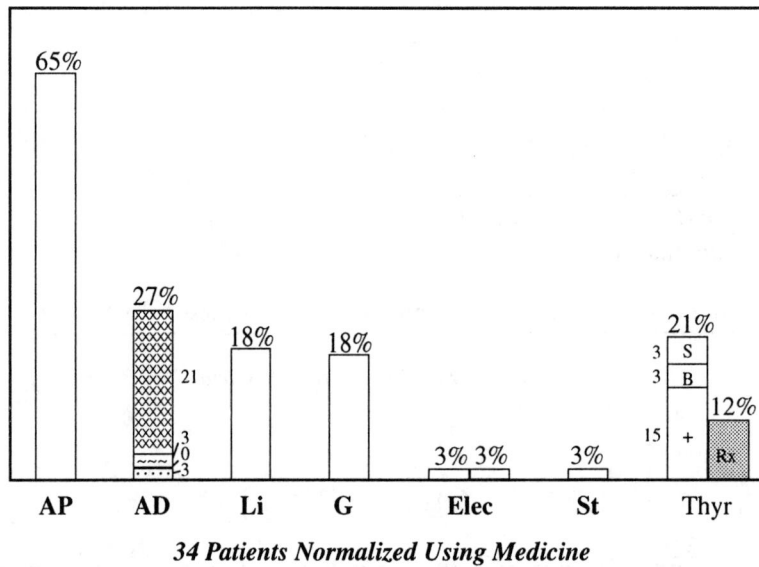

65% 27% 18% 18% 3% 3% 3% 21% 12%

21
3
0
3

3
3
15

S
B
+
Rx

AP   AD   Li   G   Elec   St   Thyr

34 Patients Normalized Using Medicine

Blends in 29%

HYPERACTIVITY HISTORY

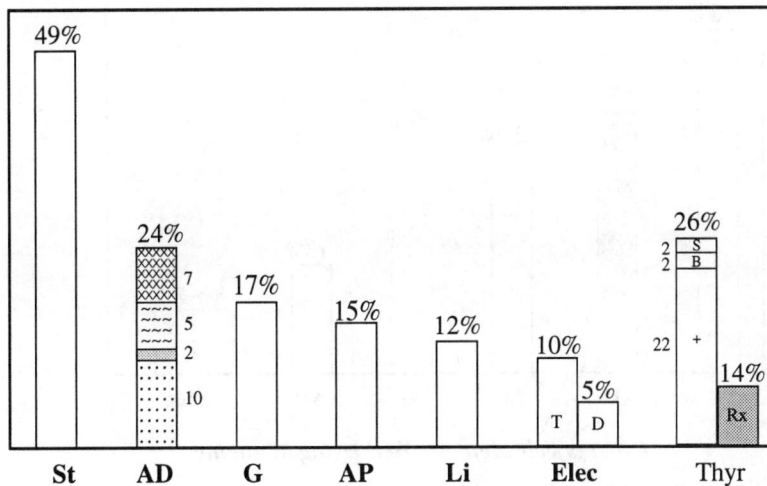

41 Patients Normalized Using Medicine

Blends in 37%

If Wellbutrin was included with stimulant percentages, the total was 59%.

Wellbutrin Resembles a Diet Pill Structurally

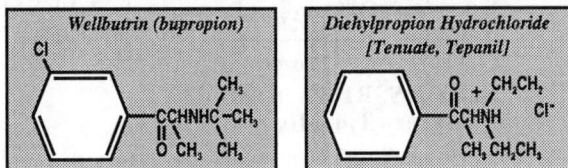

Stimulant treatment 25% of the time required a low dose of neuroleptic which was not recorded in the graph.

T H Y R O I D
M A L F U N C T I O N

97% Hypothyroid: (Lab + in the present or distant past)

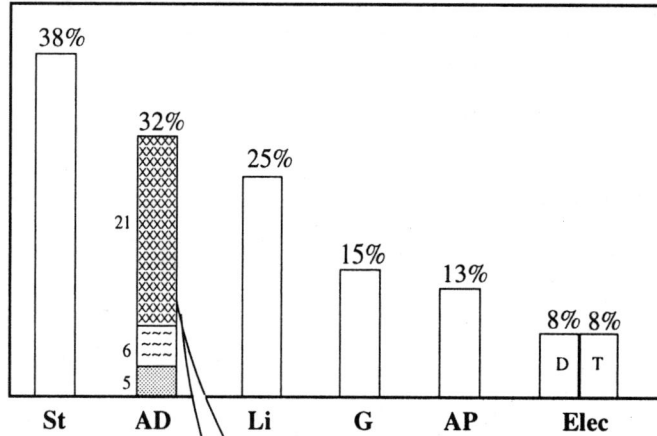

40 Patients Felt Mentally Well Using Medicine

Blends in 40%

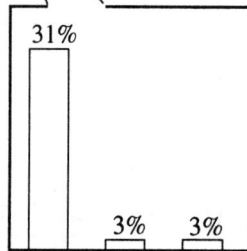

Zoloft Paxil Prozac

**AMONG SSRI'S ZOLOFT
HELPED THE MOST**

Stimulant treatment required a low dose of antipsychotic in 13%, which was not recorded in the graph.

Occasionally thyroid medicine alone worked, but usually not. 83% were on thyroid replacement medicine.

F A T I G U E

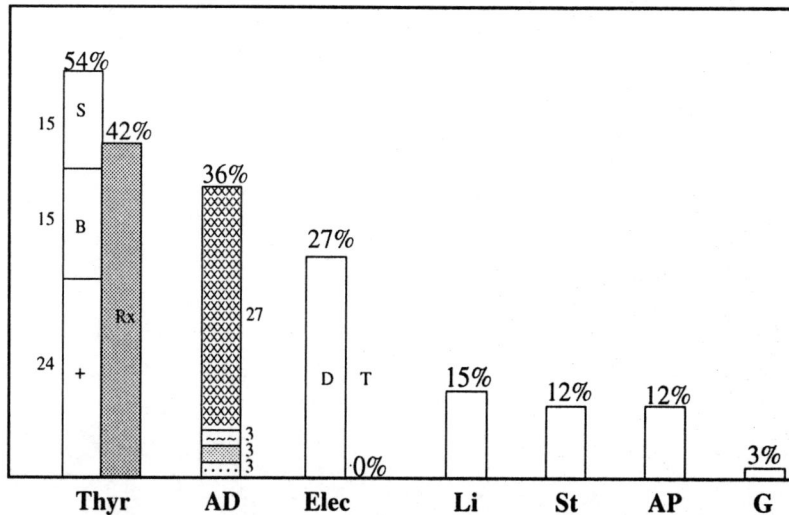

34 Patients Normalized Using Medicine

Blends in 38%

Stimulant treatment 25% of the time required a low dose of neuroleptic which was not recorded in the graph.

ALCOHOLISM

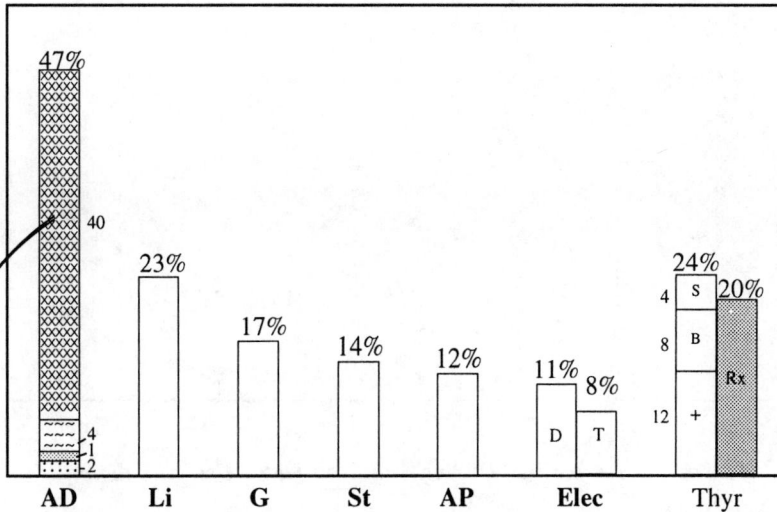

90 Patients Normalized During And After Detox Using Medicine
Blends in 38%
Stimulant treatment required a low dose of neuroleptic 14% of the time,
which was not recorded in the graph.

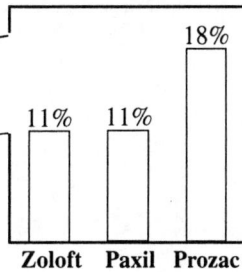

SEDATIVE HYPNOTIC ADDICTION

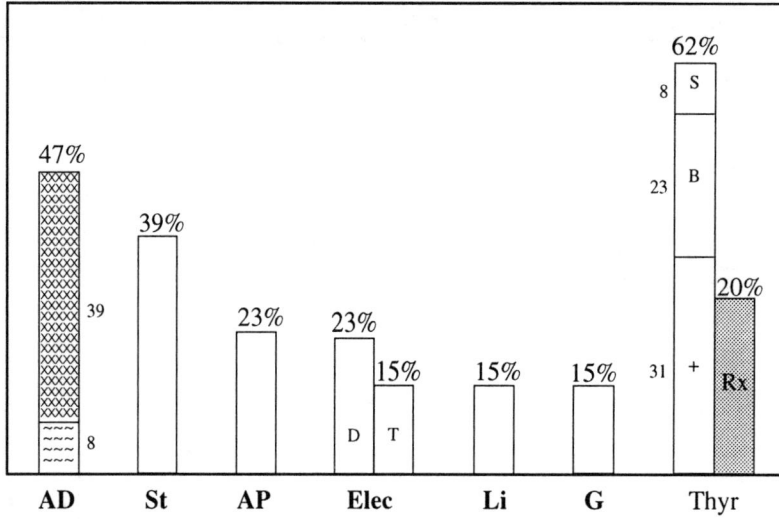

Bar chart with categories: AD, St, AP, Elec, Li, G, Thyr

- AD: 47% (39 / 8)
- St: 39%
- AP: 23%
- Elec: 23% (D), 15% (T)
- Li: 15%
- G: 15%
- Thyr: 62% (S 8 / B 23 / + 31), 20% (Rx)

13 Patients Normalized During And After Detox Using Medicine
Blends in 69%
Stimulant treatment required a low dose of antipsychotic 21% of the time,
which was not recorded in the graph.

HEROIN/OPIATE ADDICTION

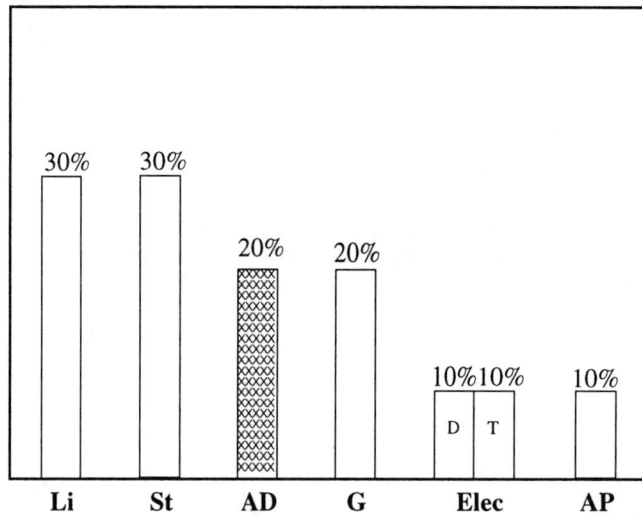

Bar chart with categories: Li, St, AD, G, Elec, AP

- Li: 30%
- St: 30%
- AD: 20%
- G: 20%
- Elec: 10% (D), 10% (T)
- AP: 10%

10 Patients Normalized During And After Detox Using Medicine
Blends in 30%

COCAINE OR AMPHETAMINE DEPENDENCE

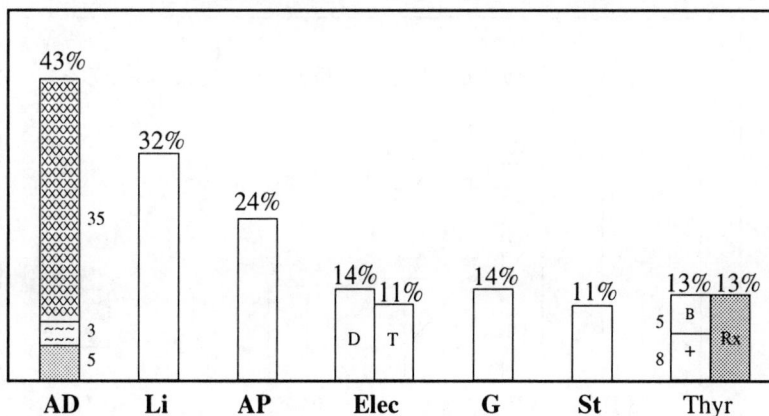

43%
35
3
5
AD

32%
Li

24%
AP

14% 11%
D   T
Elec

14%
G

11%
St

13% 13%
5   B
8   +   Rx
Thyr

37 Patients Normalized During And After Detox Using Medicine

Blends in 30%

MARIJUANA DEPENDENCE

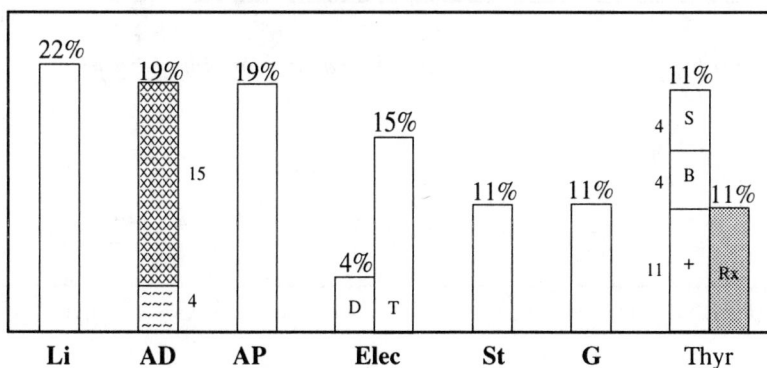

22%
Li

19%
15
4
AD

19%
AP

15%
4%
D   T
Elec

11%
St

11%
G

11%
4   S
4   B
11   +
11%
Rx
Thyr

27 Patients Felt Improvement Using Medicine

Blends in 26%
Stimulant treatment required a low dose of neuroleptic 36% of the time,
and was not recorded in the graph.

CIGARETTES - NICOTINE

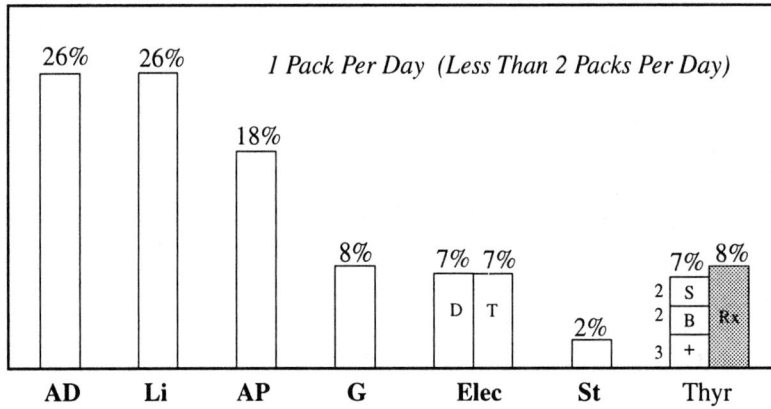

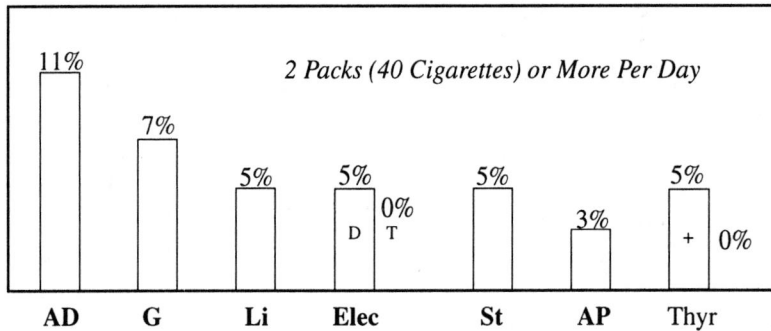

1 Pack Per Day (Less Than 2 Packs Per Day)

26%	26%	18%						
			8%	7% 7%			7%	8%
				D T			2 S	
							2 B	Rx
					2%		3 +	
AD	**Li**	**AP**	**G**	**Elec**	**St**		**Thyr**	

Blends in 16%

CIGARETTES - NICOTINE

2 Packs (40 Cigarettes) or More Per Day

11%						
	7%					
		5%	5% 0%	5%		5%
			D T		3%	+ 0%
AD	**G**	**Li**	**Elec**	**St**	**AP**	**Thyr**

Blends in 10%

Stimulant treatment required a low dose of antipsychotic 28% of the time, which was not recorded in the graph.

A Total Of 62 Patients Were Helped By Medicine

C O F F E E   E X C E S S

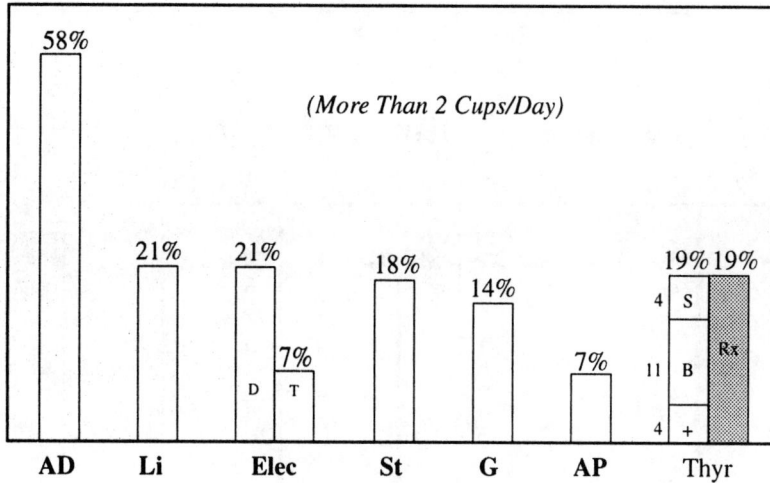

(More Than 2 Cups/Day)

58% AD
21% Li
21% D / 7% T Elec
18% St
14% G
7% AP
19% (4 S, 11 B, 4 +) / 19% Rx Thyr

28 Patients Were Comforted
(Medicine Was For Other Serious Problems)

Blends in 46%
Stimulant treatment required a low dose of neuroleptic 22% of the time,
which was not recorded in the graph.

C R E A T I V I T Y

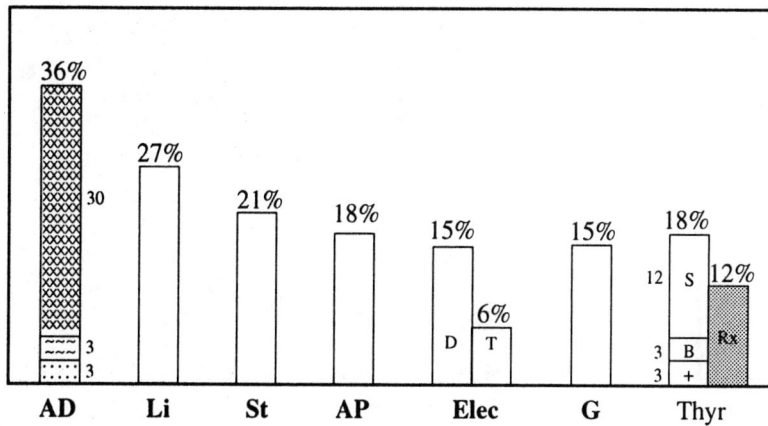

36% (30, 3, 3) AD
27% Li
21% St
18% AP
15% D / 6% T Elec
15% G
18% (12 S, 3 B, 3 +) / 12% Rx Thyr

33 Patients Were Comforted
(Medicine Was For Other Serious Problems)

Blends in 39%
Stimulant treatment required a low dose of neuroleptic 43% of the time,
which was not recorded in the graph.

CHEMICAL IMBALANCE "FOOTPRINTS"
(A RUDIMENTARY SKETCH OF ATTENTION DEFICIT DISORDERS VERSUS MANIC DEPRESSION)

A Medication Reactions Profile Can Be Used As A Clue For Which System Is Disturbed.

PROTOCALS: I   II   III   IV   V

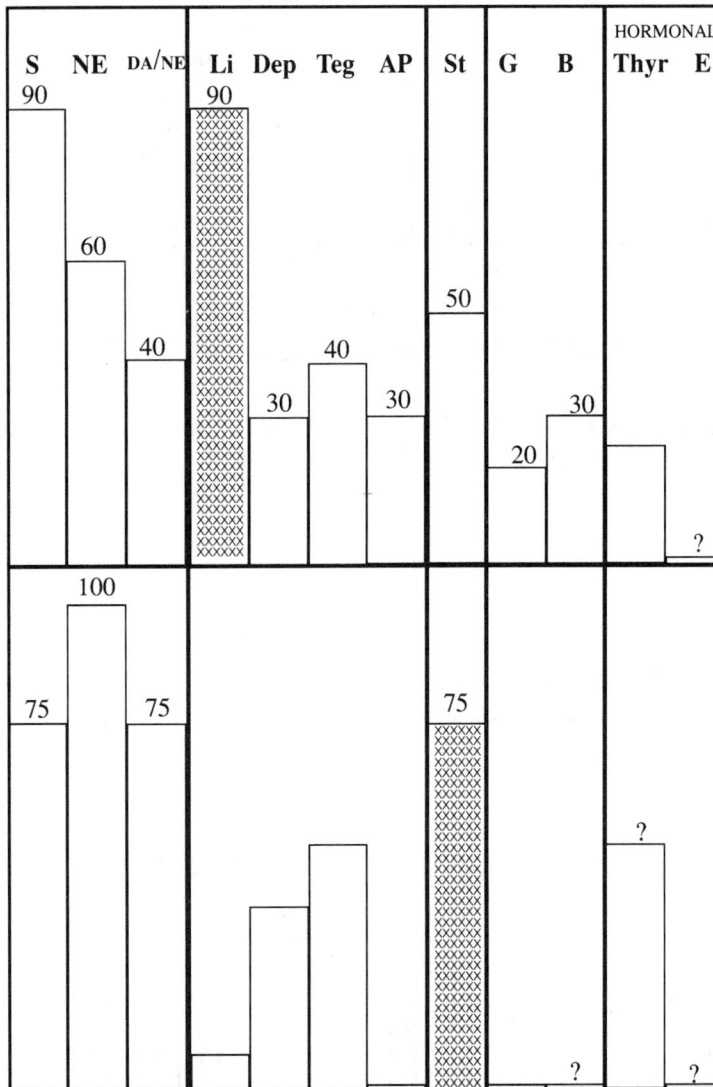

Columns / labels (left to right):
1. S
2. NE
2. DA/NE
3. Li
4. Dep
4. Teg
5. AP
6. St
7. G
8. B
9. Thyr (HORMONAL)
10. E

Percentages of Adverse Medication Reactions in Attention Deficit Disorder Patients (Chemical Failure)

S 90 · NE 60 · DA/NE 40 · Li 90 · Dep 30 · Teg 40 · AP 30 · St 50 · G 20 · B 30 · Thyr ? · E ?

Percentages of Adverse Medication Reactions in Manic Depressive Patients (Chemical Instability)

S 75 · NE 100 · DA/NE 75 · St 75 · Thyr ? · (others ?)

Ideas on why, in attention deficit disorders many substances may cause antagonism or irritation of failed DA/NE sites

1. S - Sitebinding, no action
2. NE - Sitebinding, limited action
   DA/NE - sitebinding, action sometimes
3. Li - Irritation of organicly injured site?
4. Dep - Flattens already low DA/NE/Electrical system
   Teg - Binds site, no action (has structure of NE A.D.) - and flattens electricity further
5. AP - lowers DA in failed DA/NE system
6. St - sitebinding, action, versus mismatch and no action
7. G - inhibits failed DA/NE systems
8. B - Lowers NE further

Chemical instability and chemical failure frequently coexist, making treatment difficult. Lithium worsens one and stimulant worsens the other.
One condition is usually predominant.

Severe GABA Failure — Infrequent, resembles ADHD profile (adverse reactions in all categories except GABA)

for the physician

DOSAGE TABLES

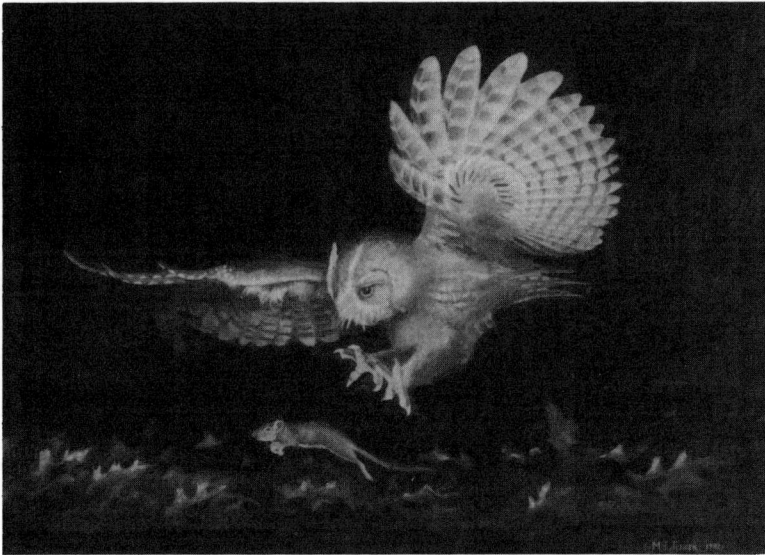

An aggressive "go get it" attitude concerning chemical imbalance gets the job done.

ANTIDEPRESSANTS

CHEMICAL	BRAND NAMES	INITIAL DOSAGE PER DAY Starting	Elderly receive half this Max. mg.	Brain Transmitter Effects (*1) S %	NE %	DA %	PEAK Concentration in Hours	HALF LIFE in Hours	Sedation (see #3)	Anticholinergic (Dry Mouth)	Orthostatic BP (Dizzy)	Cardiac Effect	Seizure Risk	Weight Gain	C=Capsule Sizes / T=Tablet Sizes / L=Liquid Concentrate / IM=Intramuscular Shot / Scored tablets underlined
SSRI's SNRI															
Sertraline	ZOLOFT	50 mg in a.m.	200	100	0	0	6	26	0	0	0	+/-	0/1	0/-	T-50, 100 mg
Paroxetine	PAXIL	20 mg in a.m	50	100	0	0	5	24	0	0	0	+/-	0/1	0/-	T-20, 30 mg
Venlafaxine	EFFEXOR	37.5mg 7 a.m 5p.m.	375	100	33	0	1.5	8	0	0	0	+/-	1	0/-	T-25, 37.5, 50, 75, 100 mg
Fluvoxamine	LUVOX	50 mg	300	100	0	0	5	16	0	0	0	+/-	2	0/-	T-50, 100
Fluoxetine	PROZAC	20 mg in a.m.	80	100	0	0	7	216 (9 days)	0	0	0	+/-	1	0/-	C-10, 20 mg; L-20mg / 5ml (120ml)
TRICYCLICS & OTHERS															
Nefazodone	SERZONE	100 mg2x/day	600	+	+	0	1	3	3	+/-	1	1	1	+/0	T-100, 150, 200, 250mg
Trazodone	DESYREL	50-75 mg HS	600	100	0	0	1.5	6	2	3	2	1	1	1	T-50, 100, 150, 300 mg
Clomipramine	ANAFRANIL	25mg HS	250	100	33	0	4	96	3	3	3	3	3	2	C-25, 50, 75 mg
Amitriptyline	ELAVIL / ENDEP	25-50mg HS	300	33	33	0	7	22	3	3	3	3	2	2	T-10, 25, 50, 75, 100, 150 mg; IM-10mg/ml
Perphenazine/Amitriptyline	TRIAVIL ETRAFON	2/25-4/50 HS 2/25-4/25 HS	16/200 32/200	33	33	Lower									T-2/10, 2/25, 4/10, 4/25, 4/50 HS; T-2/10, 2/25, 4/25
Doxepin	SINEQUAN/ ADAPIN	25-50mg HS	300	16	33	0		17	3	2	3	2	2	1	C-10, 25, 50, 75, 100, 150 mg; L-10mg/ml (120ml) Sinequan only
Trimipramine	SURMONTIL	25-50mg HS	300	16	33	0		10	3	3	2	3	2	1	C-25, 50, 100 mg
Imipramine	TOFRANIL	25-50 mg HS 25mg IM, 2X/Day	300 100 IM	33	33	0	1.5	25	2	2	2	2	2	1	T-10, 25, 50 mg; C-Tofranil PM-75, 100, 125, 150 mg; IM-25mg/2ml
Nortriptyline	PAMELAR	25mg HS	150	16	66	0		32	1	1	+/-	2	2	1	C-10, 25, 50, 75; L-10mg/5ml (16 oz)
Protriptyline	VIVACTIL	5mg-3X/Day	60	16	66	0		78	1	2	1	3	2	1	T-5, 10
Amoxapin	ASCENDIN	25mg-2X/Day	400	16	66	Lower	1.5	8	1	1	2	2	2	+/0	T-25, 50, 100, 150 mg
Maprotiline	LUDIOMIL	25-50mgHS	225	0	66	0	12	51	2	2	2	2	3	1	T-25, 50, 75 mg
Desipramine	NORPRAMINE	25mg in A.M	300	15	100	0		22	2	1	1	2	1	+/0	T-10, 25,50,75,100,150
Bupropion	WELLBUTRIN	A.M. Noon	150 3X/Day	0	0	16 (*2)	2	14	1-	0	0	+/-	4	0/-	T-75, 100
MONAMINE OXIDASE INHIBITORS							Discontinue for 14 days before starting antidepressant, buspar, stimulant or thyroid								DANGEROUS IF DIETARY RESTRICTIONS ARE NOT FOLLOWED
Phenelzine	NARDIL	increase rapidly as tolerated until well, then reduce		66	66	66			1+,1-	0	3	0	0	+/-	T-15
Tranylcypromine	PARNATE	increase by 10mg weekly		66	66	66			1-	0	3	0	0	+/0	T-10

(*1) – Since the serotonin and NE systems are highly interdependent, serotonin antidepressants also increase NE. Different antidepressants though can have different overall effects. (Manic Depressive Illness, Goodwin, Jamison, 1990, page 418).

(*2) – Structurally resembles a stimulant   •(*3) – Sedation with these medicines often indicates a protocol 2 or 3 chemistry is present   • HS = Hour of sleep (bedtime)

MOOD STABILIZERS

	STARTING DOSAGE	PEAK CONCETRATION	HALF LIFE	T-Tablet SIZES C=capsule sizes L=Liquid concentrate scored tablets underlined
LITHIUM CARBONATE SLOW RELEASE **ESKALITH CR** SLOW RELEASE **LITHOBID**	1/2 - 1 tablet: 2 X/day 1 tablet, 2 X/day	4-6 hrs	22 hrs (range 17-36 hrs)	T-450 mg T-300 mg
LITHIUM CARBONATE **ESKALITH**	1 capsule or tablet 2 or 3X/day	1/2-2 hrs	22 hrs	C-300 mg T-300 mg
LITHONATE LITHOTABS	1 capsule 2 or 3 X/day 1 tablet 2 or 3 X/day			C-300 mg T-300 mg
LITHIUM CARBONATE	150-300 mg: 2 or 3 X/day			C-150,300,600 mg. T-300 mg
LITHIUM CITRATE / LIQUID LITHIUM CITRATE	1 tsp: 2 or 3 X/day	1/4-1 hr	22 hrs	L-300 mg/tsp (5ml) 500 ml bottles
Divalproex **DEPAKOTE**	125 mg: 1-2 capsules or tablets 3 X/day	3-4 hrs	11 hrs (range 6-16 hrs)	C-sprinkle capsules 125 mg T-125, 250, 500 mg
Carbamazepine **TEGRETAL**	100 mg: 2 or 3 X/day 1 tsp: 2 or 3 X/day	4-5 hrs 1.5 hrs	15 hrs (initially 25-65 hrs)	T-100 / 200 mg L-100 mg/tsp (5ml) 450 ml bottles
Gabapentin **NEURONTIN**	100 mg 3 X/day		6 hrs	C-100, 300 mg
Clonazepam **KLONOPIN** (Similar to Ativan (a benzodiazepine) but a weak seizure medicine.	0.5-1mg at bedtime or twice daily	1-2 hrs	23 hrs (18-20)	T-0.5, 1, 2 mg
Propranolol **INDERAL**	20 mg (1/2-1): 3 or 4 X/day	1-1.5 hrs	4 hrs	T-10, 20, 40, 60, 80 mg

ANTIPSYCHOTICS

CHEMICAL	BRAND NAMES	INITIAL DOSAGE PER DAY (Starting)	Max. mg	EQUIVALENT ORAL DOSE	EPS (Muscle Cramps, Restlessness, Shuffling)	SEDATION	ANTICHOLINERGIC (Dry Mouth)	ORTHOSTATIC BP (Dizzy)	CLASS	Notes (ORAL - Peaks in 2-4 hours; Half Life - 20-40 hours; IM - Peaks in 30-60 minutes; 3-4 X more potent than oral)	Sizes (C=Capsule Size, T=Tablet Sizes, L=Liquid Concentrate, IM=Intramuscular Shot, Scored tablets underlined)
Risperidone	RISPERDAL	1mg:twice day 1 / 2mg twice day 2 / 3mg twice day 3	4-6mg/day maximum:16mg	1 mg	1	1	1	3	A		T-1,2,3,4mg
Haloperidol	HALDOL	0.5-5mg:3 X/day OR / 2-5mg:IM hourly	100mg / 25mg	3mg / 2mg	5	2	1	1	B	ideal for rapid control of severe psychosis, least painful IM shot	T-0.5,1,2,5,10,20 mg; L-2mg/ml (15ml,120ml,240ml); IM-5mg/ml
Fluphenazine	PROLIXIN	1-2.5mg:3or4 X/day OR / 1.25mg IM:3or4 X/day	40mg / 10mg	2mg	5	2	2	2	C	IM more painful than Haldol IM	T-1,2.5,5,10mg; L-2.5mg/5ml (60ml,473ml); IM-2.5mg/ml
Thiothixene	NAVANE	2-5mg:3 X/day OR	60mg	5mg	4	2	2	2	D		C-1,2,5,10,20mg; L-5mg/ml (120ml: 2-10mg dropper)(30ml: 2-5mg dropper); IM-2mg/ml, 5mg/ml
Trifluoperazine	STELAZINE	4mg IM:2-4 X/day OR	30mg / 50mg	5mg	4	1	2	2	C	Potent and not sedating	T-1,2,5,10mg; L-10mg/ml (60ml); IM-2mg/ml
Perphenazine	TRILAFON	1-2mg IM every 4 hours / 4-8mg:3 X/day OR / 5-10mg IM OR / 1mg IV every minute, a maximum of 5 times	10mg / 64mg / 16mg	8mg	4	2	2	2	C		T-2,4,8,16mg; L-16mg/5ml (118ml); IM/IV-5mg/ml
Pimozide	ORAP	1mg: 1 or 2 X/day	0.2mg/kg/day or 10mg whichever is less	1mg		2	2	2	E	for tourettes, but cardiac toxic risk (Prolonged QT interval)	T-2mg
Molindone	MOBAN	5-15mg: 3 or 4 X/day	225mg	10mg	4	2	2	2	F	can help weight loss but has more neurotoxicity, seizure risk	T-5,10,25,50,100mg; L-20mg/ml (120ml)
Loxapine	LOXITANE	5-10mg:2 X/day OR / 12.5-50mg:IM 2-4X/day	250mg / 5 days	12mg	3	3	2	3	G	only 2% gain weight	C-5,10,25,50mg; L-25mg/ml (120ml); IM-50mg/ml
Chlorprothixene	TARACTIN	25-50mg: 3 or 4 X/day oral or IM	600mg	100mg		2	2	2	D		T-10,25,50,100mg; L-100mg/5ml (473ml-1 pint); IM-25mg/2ml
Mesoridazine	SERENTIL	25-50mg:3 X/day OR / 25mg IM every 30-60 min.	100-400mg/day / 200 mg/day	50mg	2	4	4	4	H	similar to Mellaril, but injectable	T-10,25,50,100 mg; L-25mg/ml (118ml); IM-1ml (25mg)
Chlorpromazine	THORAZINE	10-25mg:3 X/day OR / 25mg IM, may repeat 25-50mg in 1 hour, then every 4 hours if needed	1000mg / 2000mg rarely needed	100mg	3	4	3	4	I	good to calm violence, sedating, most likely to cause seizure at high dose	T-10,25,50,100,200mg; C-(sustained release) spansule 30,75,150mg; L-syrup 10mg/5ml (120 ml) or concentrate 30mg/ml (118ml); 100mg/ml (236ml); IM/IV 25mg/ml (1 or 2ml ampules); Suppositories - 25mg, 100mg
Thioridazine	MELLARIL	10-25mg:2-4 X/day (mild) OR / 50-100mg:3X/day (severe)	800mg	95mg	1	4	5	5	H	minimal risk for seizures, but extreme doses can cause retinal damage	T-10,15,25,50,100,150,200mg; L-30mg/ml (10,25,50mg dropper)-118ml; 100mg/ml (100,150,200mg dropper)-118ml; Mellaril-S suspension:25mg/ml or 100mg/5ml; 473ml bottle
Clozapine	CLOZARIL	25mg: 1/2 tablet 1 or 2 X/day, increase by 25-50mg/day as tolerated to 300-400mg/day in 2 weeks, then increase by 100mg, every 3-7 days up to 900 mg/day (300mg 3 X/day) if needed		80mg	0, no T.D.	5	5	4	J	Only for severe schizophrenics who do not respond. A weekly WBC count with 3,5000/mm3 is required due to Agranulocytosis risk. Seizure risk (5%-dose related), sedation and low blood pressure make a divided dose schedule important	T-25,100mg

LONG ACTING ANTIPSYCHOTIC SHOTS (DEPOT NEUROLEPTICS)

	DOSAGE	RANGE	PEAK	HALF LIFE	SIZES & CONVERSIONS
Haloperidol Decanoate HALDOL DECANOATE	No more than 100 mg IM initially, may repeat the balance in 3-7 days, then injections monthly	50-300 mg IM every 2-5 weeks	3-9 days	21 DAYS	10-20 times the daily oral dose equals the monthly Decanoate dose • 50 mg/ml • 100 mg/ml
Fluphenazine Decanoate PROLIXIN DECANOATE	12.5 - 25 mg IM every 3 weeks (0.5 - 1 ml)	6.25-100mg IM every 3-6 weeks	1-2 days	8 days	A 20 mg tablet/day equals 25 mg/ml Decanoate every 3 weeks
Fluphenazine Enanthate PROLIXIN ENANTHATE	25 mg (1 ml) IM every 2 weeks	12.5-100 mg IM every 1-3 weeks	2-4 days	4 days	• 25mg/ml vial

SIDE EFFECT MEDICINES FOR ANTIPSYCHOTICS

Stop or reduce these in several weeks to see if they are still needed

CHEMICAL	BRAND NAMES	INITIAL DOSAGE PER DAY		Muscle Cramps (Dystonia)	Restlessness (Akathisia)	Shuffling (Akinesia)	Lip Tremor (Rabbit)	Rigidity	Tremor	C=Capsule Sizes / T=Tablet Sizes / L=Liquid Concentrate / IM=Intramuscular Shot / Scored tablets underlined
		Starting	Maximum							
Biperiden	AKINETON	•1 tablet: 1-3 X/day •2mg, IM or IV every 30 minutes, up to 4 X/day	16mg 8mg	1	1	2	2	2	1	T-2mg IM/IV-5mg/ml
Trihexyphenidyl	ARTANE	•1-5mg: 3 X/day •5 mg: 1-2 X/day	15mg	2	2	2	2	2	1	T-2, 5mg L-2mg/5ml (16 oz) C-Sequels 5mg sustained release
Diphenhydramine	BENADRYL	•25-50mg: 3 or 4 X/day •25-50mg: IM or IV	300 mg children: 5mg/kg/day	2.5	2	1	2	1	2	C-25, 50mg IM/IV-10, 50 mg/ml
Benztropine	COGENTIN	•1-2mg twice daily •1-2mg IM or IV	8mg	3	2	2	2	3	2	T-0.5, 1, 2mg IM/IV-1mg/ml
Procyclidine	KEMADRIN	•1/2-1 tablet: 3X/day	20mg	2	1	2	2	2	1	T-5mg.
Amantadine	SYMMETREL	•1 capsule: twice daily •1-2 tsp: 2 or 3 X/day	300 mg	2	2	3	2	3	2	C-100mg. L-50mg/5ml
Propranolol	INDERAL	•10-20mg: 3X/day up to 40 mg: 4 X/day •1 in A.M. (Inderal LA)	160mg CAUTION can lower blood pressure	0	3	0	2	0	0	T-10, 20, 40, 60, 80 mg C-Inderal LA - 60, 80, 120 160 mg (long acting)
Diazepam	VALIUM	•5mg: 3 X/day •5-10 mg IM or IV, no faster than 5mg/minute	40mg 20mg	3	2	0	2	2	0	T-2, 5, 10mg IM/IV 5mg/ml
Lorazepam	ATIVAN	•1-2mg: 3 X/day •No faster than 2 mg/min	10mg 2mg	0	2	0	0	0	0	T-0.5, 1, 2mg IM/IV - 1, 2, 4mg/ml
Dantrolene	DANTRIUM	•50 mg: 1-4 X/day 0.8-10 mg/kg/day half life 4-8 hrs.	For Neuroleptic Malignant Syndrome							C-25, 50, 100 mg IV-20mg/70ml
Bromocriptine	PARLODEL	•7.5-60mg/day								T-2, 5mg C-5mg

CODE:
0 = no effect
1 = mild effect
2 = moderate effect
3 = excellent

ATTENTION DEFICIT DISORDER TREATMENTS

CHEMICAL	BRAND NAMES	DOSAGE PER DAY — Starting	DOSAGE PER DAY — Maximum	Peak in Hours	Half Life in Hours	Comments	C=Capsule Sizes / T=Tablet Sizes / TTS=Skin Patch / Scored tablets underline
Methylphenidate / amphetamine	RITALIN TABLET S.R.	5mg at 8 AM, noon and 4 PM / 20mg in A.M.	• 60mg / • children 2mg/kg	1.9hrs / 4.7hrs	3hrs / lasts 8 hrs	The standard to compare other ADD treatments by	T-5, 10, 20mg slow release (S.R.) - 20mg
Dextroamphetamine / amphetamine	DEXTROSTAT / DEXEDRINE TABLET / SPANSULE	children 3-5 years of age: 2.5mg in A.M. age 6 and older: 5mg at 8 A.M. and noon and perhaps 4 P.M.	• children 1mg/kg / • 40mg / rarely more	2hrs / 2hrs / 9hrs	10hrs	usually strongest	T-5, 10mg / T-5mg / C-"spansule" 5, 10, 15mg
Phentermine / diet pill - weak amphetamine	IONAMIN	15mg in A.M.	60mg		lasts 10-14 hrs	Not standard treatment. (See page 44). Structure resembles dexedrine	C-15, 30 mg
Diethylpropion / diet pill - weak amphetamine	TENUATE	25 mg at 8 A.M. and noon	75mg		6hrs	Not standard treatment (See page 44). Structure similar to Wellbutrin	T-25mg / T-controlled release 75 mg
Bupropion / antidepressant	WELLBUTRIN	75mg at 8 A.M. and 2 P.M.	150mg 3x/day	2hrs	14 hrs	Often fixes mild ADD, yet more seizure risk	T-75, 100mg
Pemoline / nonabusable	CYLERT	37.5mg in A.M. increased by 18.75mg weekly until well	• 112.5mg / • children 3mg/kg	3hrs.	12hrs	Occasionally works well / Liver toxicity in 3% of children	T-18.75, 37, 75mg chewable 37.5mg
Clonidine / blood pressure pill	CATAPRES	Slow increase or decrease by 1/2 tablet (0.05mg) per day or TTS 1 skin patch delivers 0.1mg/day for 5-7 days	1/2 tablet (0.05mg) 4 times/day	4hrs	13 hrs / 13 hrs	For aggressive, frustrated children with stimulant or alone when stimulant is inadequate / Caution: Dizziness	T-0.1, (0.2, 0.3mg) / TTS patches 1, 2, or 3 (0.1, 0.2, 0.3mg)

Dopamine reducers in low dose may be needed with any amphetamine if the results were initially good, then worsened.
Thioridazine - Mellaril - up to 3 mg/kg/day for children, (10, 15, or 25mg, 2-3 times per day) or 25-100mg sleeper for adults on stimulant.
Trifluoperazine - Stelazine - 1 or 2mg once, possibly twice daily for adults.

ANXIETY REDUCER MEDICINES

If a dose is too sedating, take less or switch medications

Geriatric dosages are generally halved due to slower elimination

C=Capsule Sizes
T=Tablet Sizes
L=Liquid Concentrate
IM=Intramuscular Shot
IV= Intravenous
Scored tablets underlined

CHEMICAL	BRAND NAMES	DOSAGE PER DAY Starting	Maximum	Peak in Hours	Half Life in Hours	Comments	Approximate Equivalencies	
Benzodiazepines for Anxiety								
Alprazolam	XANAX	.25-0.5mg 3 X/day	10mg	1-2	11	A panic disorder favorite	0.5 mg	T-0.25, 0.5, 1, 2mg
Chlordiazepoxide	LIBRIUM	• mild: 5 or 10 mg 3 X/day • severe: 20 or 25 mg 3 X/day • children (emergency): 5mg 2-4 X/day • IM or IV: 50-100 mg may repeat in 2-4 hours	300 mg	0.5-4	24 and 48	Dull feeling, excellent for detoxes some of which required 600 mg/day	10 mg	C-5, 10, 25mg; IM=100mg with 2ml IM diluent; IV-100mg with 5 ml sterile saline/water (injected slowly over 1 minute)
Clonazepam	KLONOPIN	• 0.5-1mg at bedtime or twice daily	4 mg	1-4	23	Also helpful for panic disorders, up to 20 mg/day allowed for Epilepsy	0.5mg	T-0.5, 1, 2 mg
Clorazepate	TRANXENE	• 15-30mg at bedtime or divided doses	60 mg	1-2	73	Similar to Valium, 90mg allowed in alcohol detox	7.5mg	T-3.75, 7.5, 15 mg "Tranxene T-tabs"; T-22.5mg "Tranxene S.D."; 11.25mg - "Tranxene S.D. half strength"
Diazepam	VALIUM	• 2-5mg: 2-4 X/day • children over 6 months (emergency) 1-2.5mg: 3-4 X/day, increase as needed or tolerated • IM or IV - moderate:2-5mg, repeat in 3 hours if necessary; severe: 5-10mg, repeat in 3 hrs if necessary	40mg	1.5-2	43 & 73	Euphoric, but effective	5 mg	T-2,5,10 mg; IM/IV-5mg/ml: 2ml, 10ml (IV-inject slowly at least 1 min. per 5 mg (1ml); Tel-E-Ject: 10mg/2ml injectable syringe
Lorazepam	ATIVAN	• 0.5-1mg: 2-3 X/day • IM or IV-2mg (or 0.02mg/lb or 0.044mg/kg) whichever is less	10mg	2 / IM 1-1.5 / IV 15 min	14	A panic disorder favorite	1 mg	T-0.5, 1, 2mg; IM/IV-1mg Tubex (0.5ml fill) syringe 2mg/ml, 4mg/ml vials
Oxazepam	SERAX	• mild: 10-15mg: 3-4 X/day • severe: 15-30mg:3-4X/day	120mg	3	7	Short acting; good for detox in elderly or medically ill patients	15mg	C-10,15,30mg; T-15mg
Miscellaneous Agents for Anxiety								
Ethanol	ALCOHOL	used socially	30-90 min.	14 min. but a maximum of 1 oz. (30 ml) per 3 hrs.			1/2 glass wine(?)	
Buspirone	BUSPAR	5mg: 3 X/day	60mg	40-90 min	2.5	Very gentle, may effect serotonin	15 mg	T-5, 10 mg
Beta Adrenergic Blockers for palpitations, anxiety								
Propranolol	INDERAL	40mg: 1/2-1, 3 or 4 X/day	160mg	1-1.5	4			T-10, 20, 40, 60, 80 mg
Atenolol	TENORMIN	25 mg: 1/2 - 1 once or twice daily		2-4	7	Safer if asthma, diabetes or heart failure occuring		T-25, 50, 100 mg

74

THYROID

CHEMICAL NAME	BRAND NAME	HALF LIFE	EQUIVALENCY	"SUBCLINICAL" STARTING DOSE FOR DEPRESSION	T= TABLETS SIZES mcg
T4	SYNTHROID LEVOXYL	6 Days	50mcg to 75 mcg	12.5 - 25 mcg / day	T-25, 50, 75, (88, 100, 112, 125, 150, 175, 200, 300) mcg
	LEVOTHROID LEVO-T				T-25, 50, 75, (100, 125, 150, 175) mcg T-above, (plus 200, 300) mcg
T3	CYTOMEL TRIOSTAT	2.5 Days	25 mcg	5-6.25 mcg / day	T-5, 25, 50 mcg
T4, T3 (Mixed)	ARMOUR S-P-T THYRAR THYROLAR	T4:T3 ratio is 4:1 2.5:1 7:1 4:1	1/2 grain	T3 is approximately 4 times as potent as T4	1/4, 1/2, 1, 1.5, 2, 3, 4, 5 grain 1, 2, 3, 5 grain 1/2, 1, 2 grain 1/4, 1/2, 1, 2, 3

FEMALE HORMONES

ESTROGEN - CONJUGATED	Premarin	0.3 - 2.5 mg/day
ESTRONE	Ogen	0.625 - 5 mg/day
ESTRADIOL	Estrace	1-2 mg/day
	Estraderm	0.05- 0.1 mg transdermally twice weekly
	Estradiol Valerate (depo)	10-20 mg IM every 4-6 weeks
PROGESTERON (MPA)	Provera	2.5mg/day or 10 mg/day for last 10-13 days of estrogen cycle

SEDATING SLEEPER MEDICINES

Chemical	Brand Names	Usual Bedtime Doses	Maximum	Half Life	Form
Antidepressants					
Trazadone	**Desyrel (females)**	50-150 mg	600 mg	6 hrs	T-50,100,150,300 mg
Trimipramine	**Surmontil**	25-50 mg	300 mg	10 hrs	C-25,50,100 mg
Doxepin	**Sinequan**	10-50mg	300 mg	17 hrs	C-10, 25, 50, 75, 100, 150 mg
Amitriptyline	**Elavil** **Endep**	10-50mg	300 mg	22 hrs	T-10, 25, 50, 75, 100 ,150 mg
Imipramine	**Tofranil**	10-100 mg	300 mg	25 hrs	T-10, 25, 50 mg C-"PM" - 75, 100, 125, 150 mg
Nortriptyline	**Pamelar**	10-50 mg	150 mg	32 hrs	C-10, 25, 50, 75 mg
Mood Stabilizers					
Divalproex	**Depakote**	500-1000	(sometimes works)	11 hrs	T-125, 250, 500 mg
Carbamazepine	**Tegretal**	100-400 mg		15 hrs	T-100, 200 mg
Lithium	**Eskalith**	600 mg	(sometimes works, but singular large doses are more kidney toxic)	22 hrs	C-300 mg
Antipsychotics					
Thioridazine	**Mellaril**	10-50 mg			T-10, 15, 25, 50, 100, 150, 200 mg
Loxapine	**Loxitane**	5-30 mg			C-5, 10, 25, 50 mg
Mesoridazine	**Serentil**	10-25 mg			T-10, 25, 50, 100, 200 mg
Chlorpromazine	**Thorazine**	10-100 mg		30 hrs.	T-10, 25, 50, 100, 200 mg
or move any neuroleptic to bedtime					
Benzodiazepines (GABA)					
Zolpidem	**Ambien**	5-10 mg		2.6 hrs	T-5, 10 mg - very gentle
Triazolam	**Halcion**	0.125-0.5 mg		3.5 hrs	T-0.125, 0.25 mg
Temazepam	**Restoril**	15-30 mg		13 hrs	C-7.5, 15, 30 mg
Estazolam	**Prosom**	1-2 mg		14 hrs	T-1, 2 mg
Quazepam	**Doral**	7.5-15 mg		56 hrs	T-7.5, 15 mg
Flurazepam	**Dalmane**	15-30 mg		74 hrs	C-15, 30 mg
or move any GABA medicine to bedtime, for example:					
Alprazolam	**Xanax**	0.25 - 0.5 mg		11 hrs.	T-0.25, 0.5, 1, 2 mg
Miscellaneous					
Chloral hydrate		500-1000 mg		8 hrs.	500 mg
(barbiturate like and used for sleep during heroin detoxes)					
	Melatonin	3-6 mg	20 mg		3 mg
Decongestants					
Diphenhydramine	**Benadryl**	25-50 mg	(children maximum is 5 mg/kg/day)		Liquid T, C-25, 50 mg
Hydroxyzine	**Vistaril**	50-100 mg	(children maximum is 0.6 mg/kg)		Liquid suspension C-25, 50, 100 mg

C = Capsule
T = Tablet
Scored tablets are underlined

IDEAL WEIGHT

WOMEN				MEN			
HEIGHT	**SMALL FRAME**	**MEDIUM FRAME**	**LARGE FRAME**	**HEIGHT**	**SMALL FRAME**	**MEDIUM FRAME**	**LARGE FRAME**
4'10"	102-111	109-121	118-131	5'2"	128-134	131-141	138-150
4'11"	103-113	111-123	120-134	5'3"	130-136	133-143	140-153
5'0"	104-115	113-126	122-137	5'4"	132-138	135-145	142-156
5'1"	106-118	115-129	125-140	5'5"	134-140	137-148	144-160
5'2"	108-121	118-132	128-143	5'6"	136-142	139-151	146-164
5'3"	111-124	121-135	131-147	5'7"	138-145	142-154	149-168
5'4"	114-127	124-138	134-151	5'8"	140-148	145-157	152-172
5'5"	117-130	127-141	137-155	5'9"	142-151	148-160	155-176
5'6"	120-133	130-144	140-159	5'10"	144-154	151-163	158-180
5'7"	123-136	133-147	143-163	5'11"	146-157	154-166	161-184
5'8"	126-139	136-150	146-167	6'0"	149-160	157-170	164-188
5'9"	129-142	139-153	149-170	6'1"	152-164	160-174	168-192
5'10"	132-145	142-156	152-173	6'2"	155-168	164-178	172-197
5'11"	135-148	145-159	155-176	6'3"	158-172	167-182	176-202
6'0"	138-151	148-162	158-179	6'4"	162-176	171-187	181-207

Kilograms

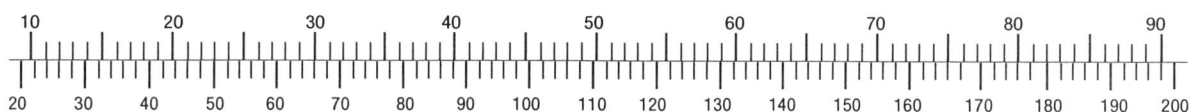

Pounds

MEDICAL ILLNESS

Checklists:

Disease Outline

As physicians, we have seen many of these conditions during our training. These medical experiences help enormously to diagnose patients entering our offices. "Organicity" often contributes to, or causes, brain chemical imbalance. What follows are superficial outlines of our training experience. Treatments can be found in Current Medical Diagnosis and Treatment, (reference 5). A specialist can be contacted if indicated for the medical diagnosis you suspect or established. Some of the diseases listed I have never seen.

Anxiety: Medical Factors Checklist

Hormonal - See page 97

-Pituitary	Cushing's disease
-Thyroid	**Hyper, hypo**
-Parathyroid	Hypo (calcium low)
-Pancreas	Hypoglycemia, insulinoma, diabetes
-Adrenal	Cushing's syndrome, Addison's disease
	Pheochromocytoma
-Ovarian	Estrogen low, **premenstrual syndrome**, menopausal

Lungs Low oxygenation:

-Chronic obstructive lung disease, pneumonia, asthma, anemia

-Pulmonary embolus - abrupt pain on breathing, rapid heart and breathing rates, most clots are from deep calf veins [x-ray, perfusion scan, lung angiography]

-Carcinoid syndrome (lung or intestinal growths), coughing and wheezing, flushing, diarrhea, high serotonin - rare

Heart - Angina

-Myocardial infarction - usually chest pain [ECG, cardiac enzymes]

-Paroxysmal atrial tachycardia - abrupt, can last hours, heart rate 140-220/minute [ECG]

-Irregularity

-Mitral valve prolapse - [echo, midsystolic click while standing, perhaps late systolic murmur]

-Congestive heart failure

Liver

-Post hepatitis syndrome, page 100, 102

Kidneys

-Uremia, page 102

Substances, Medications (Most can have mental effects)

-Caffeine, marijuana, amphetamine, cocaine, amylnitrate, hallucinogen

Withdrawal Syndromes: Alcohol, barbiturates, sedative hypnotics, opiates, nicotine, caffeine

-Psychotropic medicines, page 38

-Antipsychotics (**Akathisia**) - restlessness

-Anticholinergic toxicity - dry mouth, flushed, blurring, dilated pupils, constipation (ileus)

-Antihypertensive and cardiac medicines (Digitalis - nausea, vomiting, headache, visual symptoms, disorientation)

-Sympathomimetics (**decongestants**), theophylline

-Aspirin intolerance, penicillin, sulfonamides

-Toxins - heavy metals, page 103

Brain

-Trauma - post concussion syndrome, page 103

-Cerebrovascular disease (stroke, hemorrhage), transient ischemic attack

-Epilepsy - (temporal lobe especially), page 102

-Migraine

-Infections - mononucleosis, viral, neurosyphilis, encephalitis, fever, page 100

-Cancer, mass, page 95

-Degenerative - Wilson's, Huntington's disease, page 96

-Meniere's disease - hearing loss, ringing, vertigo (environment spinning)

Inflammatory Disorders, page 101

-Multiple sclerosis

-Systemic lupus erythematosus, rheumatoid arthritis, polyarteritis nodosa, temporal arteritis

-Anaphylaxis - medication, food reactions, bee sting or ant bite causing"hives", itching, breathing difficulty and shock

Other

-Systemic cancer, page 95

-Electrolyte disturbances, high potassium

-Hypothermia

-Vitamin deficiencies (thiamine, folate, B_{12}, niacin), page 103

-Porphyria, page 102

Depression: Medical Factors Checklist

Hormonal - hypo or hyper functioning. See page 97.
  -Pituitary
  -**Thyroid**
  -Parathyroid
  -Adrenal, hyperaldosteronism
  -Ovarian:
  -Premenstrual   -moodiness, appetite change, breast tenderness, fluid retention, headaches
  -Postpartum   -estrogen/progesterone falling,yet this hormonal treatment fails.
  -**Menopause**   -estrogen low
Metabolic
  -Electrolytes - low potassium or sodium (diuretic induced), page 102
  -Liver encephalopathy - see page 102
  -Oxygen low
        -anemia (severe)
        -arteriosclerosis (cerebral)
        -cardiac irregularity
        -congestive heart failure
        -myocardial infarction
        -bronchitis (chronic)
        -pneumonia
        -emphysema
        -sleep apnea - usually obese middle aged male, hypertensive, loud cyclic snoring,
              daytime fatigue
  -Kidney failure, urinary tract (uremia), page 102
Drugs and Medications (most medicines can have mental effects)
  -**Alcohol**, barbiturates, sedative-hypnotics
  -**Amphetamines** (and their withdrawal)
  -Antabuse (disulfiram)
  -**Psychotropic medicines,** page 38
  -Antihypertensive and cardiac medicines (Digitalis)
  -Oral contraceptives
  -Steroids, nonsteroidal   analgesics/anti-inflammatory
  -Antibacterials (Ampicillin), antifungals
  -Chemotherapy for cancer, tagamet (Cimetidine)
  -insecticides
Vitamin Deficiency page 103
  -Thiamine - (often with alcoholism)
  -B_{12} (pernicious anemia-autoimmune)
  -Folate
  -Niacin (Pellagra)
  -Vitamin C
  -Malabsorption conditions
Infections, page 100
  -Viral: **influenza**, pneumonia, **mononucleosis**, chronic fatigue syndrome
  -**Bacterial**
  -AIDS, neurosyphili
  -**Tuberculosis, fungi**
  -Encephalitis, meningitis
  -Creutzfeldt-Jacob (dementia)
Inflammatory, page 101
  -**Multiple sclerosis**
  -Myasthenia gravis
  -**Systemic lupus erythematosus**, rheumatoid arthritis, temporal arteritis, Sjogren's arteritis

Depression: Medical Factors Checklist

Cancer (especially if major weight loss), page 95
- -Metastasis to brain
- **-Gastrointestinal**
- **-Pancreas** - also has remote effect from the primary site
- -Prostate
- -Breast
- -Lung

Brain
- -Tumor, page 95
- **-Head trauma** (concussion), page 103
- -Epilepsy (partial complex temporal lobe especially on right), page 102
- **-Stroke** (cerebrovascular disease) especially anterior hemisphere, depression first two years after stroke more likely
- -Migraines
- -Narcolepsy
- -Hydrocephalus (normal pressure), page 103
- -Degenerative Dementias: **Alzheimer's**, Pick's disease, page 96
    Parkinson's disease -50-75% depressed
    Huntington's chorea,
    Wilson's Disease,
    Fahr's disease -calcification of basal ganglia causing Parkinson symptoms,psychosis, dementia
    Olivopontocerebellar degeneration, page 91
    Amyotrophic lateral sclerosis (ALS), page 91
    Klinefelter's (XXY), page 102
- **-Endometriosis** can spread to the brain and even cause seizures.

Other
- -Porphyria, postoperative mood disorders, page 102

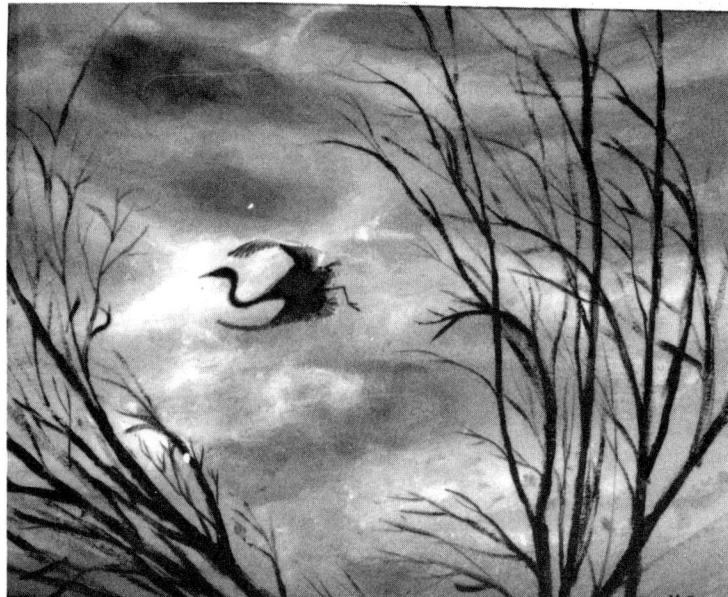

Fatigue: Medical Factors Checklist

Infection, page 100
- **Viral syndromes**
- **Mononucleosis**
- Hepatitis
- Pharyngitis
- Endocarditis
- Urinary tract infections
- Tuberculosis

Hormonal, page 97
- **Thyroid malfunction**

Toxicity
- **Medication side effects,** page 38
- Alcohol and drug abuse
- Chronic poisoning

Metabolic
- Low potassium
- Low blood sugar
- Diabetes
- **Starvation or dieting**
- **Obesity**

Cancer, page 95
- Occult malignancy
- Leukemia -WBC's high or low
- Lymphoma - tumor-like proliferation of lymphnodes and spleen
- Carcinoma of the colon

Vascular conditions
- Atherosclerotic heart disease
- Hypertension
- Rheumatic heart disease
- **Congestive heart failure**
- **Mitral valve prolapse**
- Heart disease

Lung conditions
- Asthma /chronic obstructive pulmonary disease
- Allergic disorders
- Restrictive lung diseases
- Sleep apnea

Other Conditions
- **Anemia, iron deficiency**
- B_{12} deficiency
- Pregnancy
- Systemic lupus erythematosus, page 101
- Arthritis

Hormonal, page 97

    -Thyroid: **hyperthyroid**

    -Adrenal: Cushing's disease

    -Ovarian: menses related, postpartum

    -Carcinoid (serotonin tumor), page 80

Drugs / Medications (most can have a variety of mental effects), page 38

    -**Cocaine, amphetamines**, hallucinogens,opiates, steroids

    -**Antidepressants, Tegretal (carbamepazine),** Antabuse (disulfiram), thyroid medicine

    -Levodopa, **sympathomimetics (decongestants)**

    -Chemotherapy (Procarbazine), Isoniazid for tuberculosis

    -Yohimbine, Tagamet (cimetadine) for ulcers

Infection, page 100

    -AIDS

    -Neurosyphilis

    -Encephalitis

    -Viral illness, influenza

Brain

    -Epilepsy - **Partial complex** (temporal lobe), page 102

    -Trauma (concussion), page 103, thalamotomy

    -Stroke (infarct, hemorrhage)

    -Migraines

    -Cancer, page 95 - diencephalic and third ventricle

    -Degenerative: page 96- Parkinson's (postencephalitic),

                   Huntington's, Pick's diseases

                   Fahr's disease -calcification of basal ganglia, causing Parkinson's

                       symptoms, psychosis, dementia

                   Wilson's disease

    -Klein-Levin syndrome - hypersomnic attacks for up to 2 days, 3-4 times per year with

          overeating,oversexuality, irritability, usually in young males

    -Klinefelter's - (XXY), page 99

Inflammatory, page 101

    -Multiple sclerosis

    -Sydenham's chorea - irritability and uncontrollable movements usually in children (5-15 yrs.)

          months after carditis due to streptococcal rheumatic fever

    -Systemic lupus erythematosus

Vitamin Deficiency, page 103

    -Thiamine, B_{12}, folate, niacin, C

SEASONAL SUNLIGHT SENSITIVITY WITH MANIC DEPRESSIVE CHEMISTRY

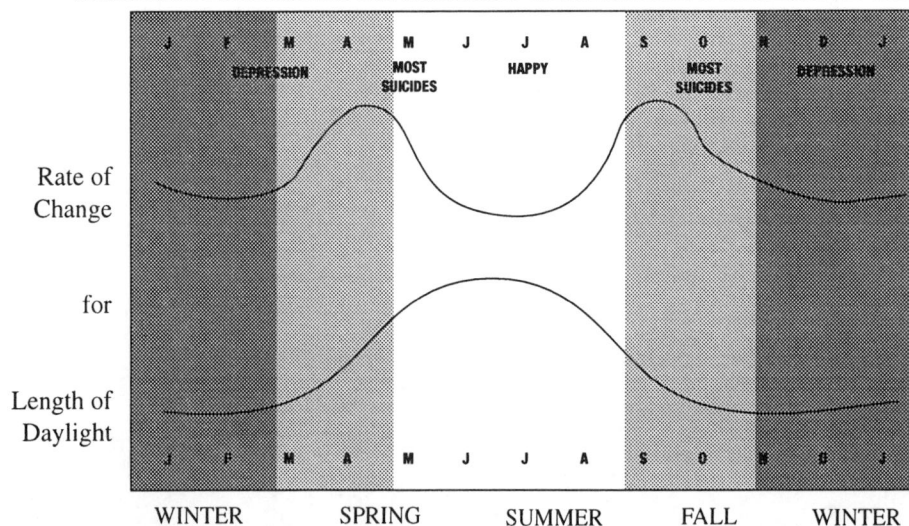

Psychosis (Bizarreness): Medical Factors Checklist

Substance induced
- **Alcohol**, **amphetamines**, amphetamine like substances, cocaine, hallucinogens (LSD, PCP, mescaline), inhalants, marijuana
- **Medications**: anticholinergic, antidepressant, antihypertensive, antiparkinson, antituberculosis, cimetadine (Tagamet), disulfiram (Antabuse), stimulant, phenobarbital, page 38
- **Withdrawal states**: **Alcohol**, barbiturate, sedative hypnotic

Delirium
Brain
- **Cancer,** page 95
- **Cerebrovascular** disease (atherosclerosis or **stroke**) -especially right brain
- **Trauma** - especially frontal or limbic lobes, page 103
- **Hydrocephalus** (normal pressure), page 103
- **Epilepsy** - especially temporal lobe, page 102
- **Degeneration,** page 96-   **Alzheimer's**
      Pick's
      Huntington's
      Parkinson's
      Wilson's
      Fahr's
      Olivopontocerebellar, page 91
      Hallervorden-Spatz disease, page 91
- **Infection,** page 100 -   Neurosyphilis
      AIDS
      Herpes simplex effecting temporal lobes (focal encephalitis)
      Creutzfeldt-Jacob

Hormonal, page 97
- **Adrenal** (Addison's, Cushing's)
- **Thyroid**
- **Parathyroid**

Metabolic
- Low blood sugar
- Low oxygen
- High calcium, page 98, 105
- **liver failure,** page 102
- **kidney failure** (uremia), page 102
- Fabry's - spider-like blood vessels in "bathing suit" area, burning (hands/feet/abdomen), leg swelling and retarded growth (galactoside renal failure).
- homocystinuria, cerebral lipidosis, metachromatic leukodystrophy.
- porphyria, page 102

Toxic
- Carbon monoxide, heavy metals, page 103

Vitamin Deficiency, page 103
- B_{12} (pernicious anemia) - autoimmune
- Thiamine (Wernicke-Korsakoff) - often alcoholic
- Niacin (Pellagra) - corn or alcohol diet usually
- Folate

Inflammatory, page 101
- **Systemic lupus erythematosus**
- Multiple sclerosis

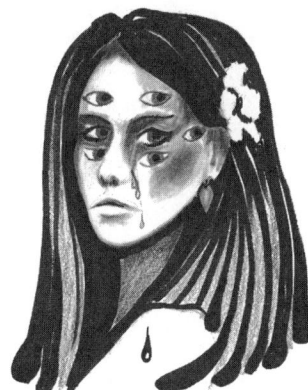

Brain

-Fetal, infantile or toddler brain stresses such as prematurity, fever, viral inflammations or head trauma.
-**Genetic heredity**
-Hidden cerebral palsy or **mental retardation**: 5-15%
-**Head trauma**, battered child syndrome, subdural hematoma, concussion, page 103
-Epilepsy - Petit mal or psychomotor seizures, page 102
-**Tourette's** - vocal and motor tics (frown, grimace, squint), familial
-**Post viral encephalitis**
-**herpes simplex may effect frontal and temporal lobes,** page 100
-**AIDS,** page 100
-**High fever injury**
-Cerebrovascular accident (**stroke**)
-Aging, growing old
-Brain tumor, page 95
-Fragile X syndrome -second most common cause of mental retardation (1 per 1-2,000): short with large long head, and large testes. Rapid perseverative talking.
-Hydrocephalus -staggering, urinary urgency / incontinence, slow, demented, page 103.

[Lab: enlarged ventricles and compressed gyri on CT / MRI, normal CSF pressure]

-Childhood Huntington's or Wilson's Disease, page 96
-Subacute sclerosing panencephalitis, page 101

Others

-Malnutrition
-**Lead intoxication** - abdominal pain, constipation, headache, irritability, wristdrop, learning disability

[Lab: blood lead level high, microcytic anemia / basophilic stippling, free erythrocyte protoporphyrin high]

-**Thyroid dysfunction,** page 97, 111
-Deafness (child "doesn't listen")

Delirium

Delirium is characterized by confusion, changing consciousness, and disorganized thinking. Memory loss, disorientation, incoherence, rambling, and hallucinations can occur. Onset is in hours or days, and fluctuates through the day.

Organic Causes of Delirium: Checklist

Withdrawal syndromes
   -Alcohol
   -Sedative Hypnotics (Xanax, Valium, etc.)
Intoxication
   -**Medications**: anticholinergics (antihistamines, tricyclic antidepressants, antipsychotics), lithium, anticonvulsants, sedative-hypnotics (Valium, etc.), alcohol, antihypertensive agents, antiarrhythmic drugs, digitalis, antiparkinsonian agents, steroids and anti-inflammatory drugs, analgesics, disulfiram (antabuse), antibiotics, antineoplastic drugs, thyroid medicine, insulin, Zantac, Tagamet.
   -**Drugs of abuse:** PCP and hallucinogenic agents (glue, nitrous oxide).
   -**Toxins:** heavy metals, organic solvents, methyl (rubbing) alcohol, ethylene glycol (antifreeze), insecticides, carbon monoxide, carbon disulfide.
Metabolic, page 102
   -Organ Failure:
      -**liver** encephalopathy
      -**kidney** and urinary tract uremia
      -**lung** hypoxia, carbon dioxide narcosis
   -**Electrolyte** imbalance: sodium, potassium, calcium, magnesium.
   -Water imbalance: inappropriate antidiuretic hormone, water intoxication, **dehydration**.
   -Acid base imbalance: acidosis, alkalosis.
   -**Hypoxia.**
   -Hypoglycemia.
   -**Cancer -remote effects**, page 95, carcinoid syndrome (rare serotonin tumor with flushing and diarrhea), page 80
   -Inborn errors of metabolism: porphyria, Wilson's disease, page 96.
   -**Vitamin** deficiency: thiamine (B_1), B_{12}, Niacin, folate, page 103.

Hormonal (Hypo or Hyper function) - see page 97
   -Thyroid
   -Parathyroid
   -Adrenal
   -Pancreas
   -Pituitary
Heart
   -Congestive heart failure (shortness of breath, ankle edema)
   -Arrhythmia
   -Myocardial infarction
Brain
   -**Head trauma,** concussion, page 103
   -**Epilepsy**, postictal states, complex partial status epilepticus, page 102
   -**Tumor** (especially frontal, temporal), subdural hematoma, abscess, aneurysm, mass (space occupying), page 95
   -**"Stroke":** thrombosis, embolism, arteritis, hemorrhage, hypertensive encephalopathy
   -**Degeneration**: Alzheimer's disease, page 96
   -**Multiple sclerosis**: Most common neurologic illness of young adults. Episodic sensory deteriorations, emotionality, optic neuritis (blindness) can occur, incontinence, unsteady gait and voice. [MRI]

Infection, page 100

      -Encephalitis, meningitis (viral, bacterial, fungal, protozoal) fever, headache, neck rigidity

      -Pneumonia,

      -Septicemia (fever, low blood pressure), Endocarditis (subacute bacterial), Influenza,

      -Mononucleosis (fatigue, sore throat, inflammation of heart, liver and brain can occur).

      -Hepatitis (flu-like, tender liver, yellow eyes / skin)

      -AIDS (sweats, diarrhea, weight loss, wasting, purple-brown skin patches (Kaposi's),

      -Neurosyphilis, (abnormal sensations, shooting pains, dementia), "gumma" lesions, muscle and
            bone pains, respiratory and cardiac distress

      -Typhoid (**Salmonella** poisoning - diarrhea, constipation,"stepladder" fever, rose spots),

      -Typhus (Rickettsia from body louse - headache, fever, trunk rash day 4-7),

      -Lyme disease (see page 100)

      -Acute rheumatic fever (Streptococcal immune process -carditis, arthritis, rash, chorea 3%),

      -Malaria (plasmodium - chills, fevers, aches),

      -Mumps (painful swollen parotids),

      -Diphtheria (corynebacterium - sore throat, myocarditis, neuropathy, seeing double, slurring, poor
            swallowing)

Blood

      -Pernicious anemia - autoimmune B_{12} malabsorption (macrocyctic anemia usually)

      -Bleeding disorders

      -Polycythemia (increased RBC mass, enlarged spleen)

Hypersensitivity

      -Serum sickness (joint pains, urticaria, fluid retention)

      -Allergic reaction

Injury

      -Temperature: hyperthermia (hot), hypothermia (cold)

      -Electricity

      -Burns

      -Post operative states

      -Body trauma

Inflammatory - see page 101

      -Systemic lupus erythematosus (SLE)

      -Temporal arteritis

      -Polyarteritis nodosa

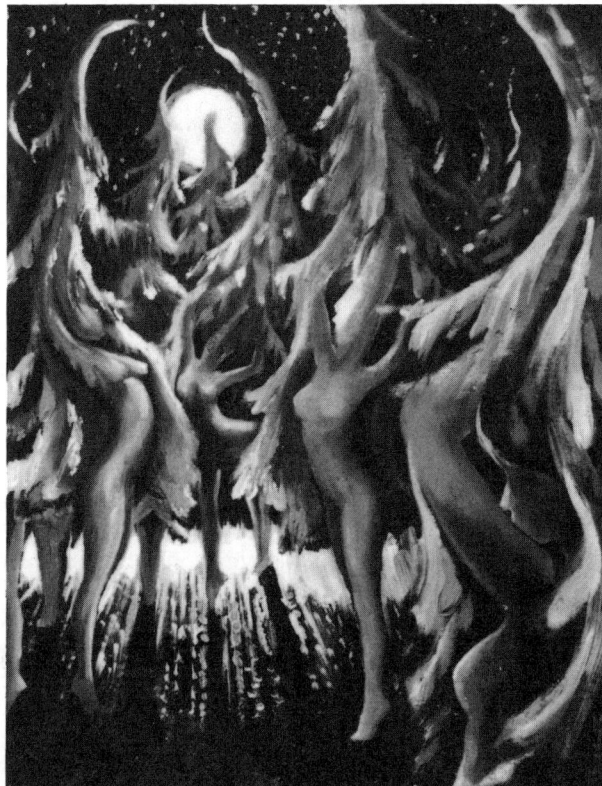

PHYSICAL EXAMINATION OF THE DELIRIOUS PATIENT

Check:	Finding	Clinical Implication
1. Pulse	Slow	Hypothyroidism Severe heart block Increased intracranial pressure
	Fast	Hyperthyroidism Infection Heart failure
2. Temperature	Fever	Sepsis Thyroid storm Vasculitis
3. Blood pressure	Low	Shock Hypothyroidism Addison's disease
	High	Encephalopathy Intracranial mass
4. Respiration	Rapid	Diabetes Pneumonia Cardiac failure Fever Acidosis (metabolic)
	Shallow	Alcohol or other substance intoxication
5. Carotid vessels	Bruits or decreased pulse	Transient cerebral ischemia
6. Scalp and face		Evidence of trauma
7. Neck	Evidence of neck rigidity	Meningitis Subarachnoid hemorrhage
8. Eyes	Papilledema	Tumor Hypertensive encephalopathy
	Pupils dilated	Anxiety Autonomic overactivity (e.g.,delirium tremens)
9. Mouth	Tongue or cheek lacerations	Evidence of generalized tonic-clonic seizures
10. Thyroid	Enlarged	Hyperthyroidism
11. Heart	Irregular	Inadequate cardiac output, possibility of emboli
	Enlarged Heart	Heart failure Hypertensive disease
12. Lungs	Congestion	Pulmonary failure Pulmonary edema Pneumonia
13. Breath	Alcohol Ketones	Diabetes
14. Liver	Enlargement	Cirrhosis Liver failure

Check:	Finding	Clinical Implication
15. Nervous system a. Reflexes-	Asymmetry with Babinski's signs	Mass lesion Cerebrovascular disease Preexisting dementia
	Snout	Frontal mass Bilateral posterior cerebral artery occlusion
b. Abducens nerve (sixth cranial nerve)	Weakness in lateral gaze	Increased intracranial pressure
c. Limb strength	Asymmetrical	Mass lesion Cerebrovascular disease
d. Autonomic	Hyperactivity	Anxiety Delirium

Adapted from table by R. L. Strub, F. W. Black:
Neurobehavioral Disorders: A Clinical Approach (1981), used with permission
F.A. Davis Company, 1915 Arch St., Philadelphia, PA, 19103

LABWORK FOR DELIRIUM

Routine choices:
- Blood chemistries: electrolytes, BUN, creatinine, glucose, liver enzymes, calcium, phosphate
- CBC with WBC differential
- Thyroid function tests (Free T_4, FTI, TSH)
- Syphilis serology
- HIV antibody test
- Erythrocyte sedimentation Rate (ESR)
- Urinalysis
- Electrocardiogram (ECG)
- Chest X-ray
- Electroencephalogram (EEG)
- Blood and urine drug screens

Additional choices:
- Blood levels of medications
- Blood, urine and CSF cultures
- Lumbar puncture and CSF examinations (protein, glucose, culture, serology, pressure)
- Serum B_{12}, folate, magnesium, ammonia, serum proteins, osmolality, arterial blood gases
- LE prep, ANA
- Urine: osmolality, porphobilinogen
- Skull film
- CT or MRI brain scan

DEMENTIA

Dementia is characterized by impaired memory, thinking and judgement, but normal consciousness without fluctuations during the course of a day.

Organic causes of Dementia Checklist:

50-60% **Alzhiemers**: incidence at age 65 is 5%, at age 85 is 25%, page 96

15-30% **Vascular Dementia** - arteriosclerotic placques, (carotid, hypertensive, diabetic)
Multiple infarcts (strokes), cortical microinfarction
Binswanger's (subcortical arteriosclerosis)
[MRI]

1-5% each **Alcoholic dementia**
Thiamine Deficiency (Wernicke-Korsakoff) - staggering neuropathy, eyes not
coordinating, page 103
Intracranial Masses: tumors, subdural mass, abscess, page 95
Head trauma, page 103
Normal pressure or obstructive **Hydrocephalus** - (staggering, incontinent), page 103

1% each AIDS, page 100
Systemic Lupus Erythematosus, collagen vascular disease, page 101
Parkinson's disease - 30% have dementia, page 96
Huntington's chorea
Progressive Supranuclear Palsy
Pick's disease -Similar to Alzheimer's, but rare, and wasting is more confined to frontal
and anterior temporal lobes. Death occurs in 2-10 years. "Pick bodies" are found
in neurons on autopsy. Language impairment is prominent. Unlike Alzheimer's,
visuospacial abilities are preserved, and memory loss occurs later.

Less than 1% Each:

Anoxia
Punch-Drunk syndrome (repeated head injury - boxers)
Neurodegenerative
Wilson's disease -See next page.
ALS (Amyotrophic lateral sclerosis) weakness, difficulty swallowing breathing, talking,
death in three years.
Spinocerebellar degenerations
Olivopontocerebellar degeneration - incoordination of walking and speech, with tremor
similar to Parkinson's
Metachromatic Leukodystrophy - granules in many organs, and demylination,
"schizophrenia", posture disturbance, progressive slight paralysis, infants to
middle aged adults effected [urine for metachromatic granules]
Hallervorden-Spatz disease -leg rigidity, jerking writhing movements, speech
incoordination. Genetic iron deposition in globus pallidus, substantia nigra.
Dementia and death before age 30
Infectious
Creutzfeldt-Jacob disease can be in adults in their 50's, and kills in 1 year. Muscle
twitches / jerks, incoordination of walking and speech, writhing in
hands, dementia, and sleepiness occur. [EEG periodic complexes]
Viral encephalitis
Progressive multifocal leukoencephalopathy, a "JC virus" opportunistic infection in the
immunocompromized causes white matter demyelination
Behcet's syndrome -small blood vessel inflammation, small recurrent ulcers of mouth,

nose, and genitalia. Can involve eye, joints, gastrointestinal and central nervous system.

Neurosyphilis, page 100

Chronic bacterial meningitis

Crytococcal meningitis, and other fungi

Nutritional, page 103

B_{12} deficiency

Folate deficiency

Niacin deficiency (Pellagra)

Marchiafava-Bignami disease - degeneration of corpus callosum due to red wine damage (healthy right arm can't move when verbal instructions given to move)

Zinc deficiency

Metabolic

Thyroid disease, page 97

Parathyroid disease, page 98

Liver failure, page 102

Kidney failure, page 102

Dialysis dementia - Long term hemodialysis can deliver aluminum and cause speech disorders, muscle jerks (myoclonic) and dementia.

Cushing's syndrome, page 99

Adrenoleukodystrophy - below

Inflammatory

Multiple Sclerosis, page 101

Whipple's disease -malabsorption, abdominal pain, diarrhea with blood, fever, arthritis, pigmentation, emaciation (bacilli in most organ systems)

Dementia Presenting in Adolescence

Wilson's Disease

Copper deposition causes hepatitis-like picture, corneal ring (green-brown), tremor, slow muscle spasms (dystonia), constant writhing movements (chorea), speech incoordination and psychosis. Autosomal recessive genetics, basal ganglia effected. [serum ceruloplasm low, 24 hour urine copper high, lower alkaline phosphatase]

Cerebral Storage Diseases (rare)

Acute Intermittent Porphyria

Intermittent abdominal pain, psychosis, neuropathy/paralysis/seizures can occur, Autosomal dominant. [High urine porphobilinogen and aminolevulinic acid during attack, sodium low]

SSPE (Subacute sclerosing panencephalitis)

In childhood, usually following measles infection or vaccination, characterized by demyelination, misbehavior, muscle jerks (myoclonus), seizures [CSF measles antibodies elevated initially, EEG - periodic complexes]

Huntington's Chorea (1 per 20,000)

Abnormal writhing movements, irritable, posturing, autosomal dominant, [CT, MRI, PET - reduced caudate nucleus]

Myoclonic Epilepsy

Adrenoleukodystrophy (Schilder's disease)

Causes loss of speech, comprehension, and coordination. Blindness, deafness, and tight spastic muscles result from massive destruction of brain white matter. Adrenals are small and their function is abnormal. X-linked recessive genetics.

92

LAB WORKUP OPTIONS FOR DEMENTIA

Chemistry Profile - SMA25
  (Serum electrolytes, glucose, calcium, liver, kidney functions)
Serum magnesium
Complete blood cell count with differential cell type count
Urinalysis
Thyroid (blood) Free T_4, FTI, TSH
Stool hemoccult for gastrointestinal bleeding, cancer
Chest X-Ray for lung cancer
RPR (serum screen), FTA-ABS (if CNS disease is suspected)
  -for syphilis
Serum B_{12}, folate
Alcohol and drug screen (blood, urine)

Erythrocyte sedimentation rate (Westergren) for vasculitis
Antinuclear antibody (ANA), C_3C_4, Anti-DS DNA for vasculitis
Arterial blood gases for hypoxia
HIV antibody test for AIDS
Urine corticosteroids (24 hours - for hyperadrenalism)
Heavy metals (blood, urine)
Urine porphobilinogens for porphyria
Urine for metachromatic granules
Serum ceruloplasm for Wilson's disease
Bromide screening if serum chloride elevated

Electrocardiogram (ECG)
Neurological workup
    CT or MRI scan of head
    SPECT for perfusion deficits
    Lumbar puncture
    EEG

Neuropsychological testing

Abnormal functioning of a nerve: burning, tingling, or weakness, longer nerves are often effected more.

Diabetes mellitus
Uremia
Nutritional
      Alcoholism, malabsorption, starvation
      Pernicious anemia (**B$_{12}$ deficiency**)
Medicines
      Vitamin B$_6$ (pyridoxine)
      INH, nitrofurantoin, antineoplastic agents
Toxins
      Nitrous oxide (anesthesia)
      Metals: lead, organic and inorganic mercury
      Organic solvents: n-hexane, toluene, and others
Infectious / inflammatory
      Vasculitis: systemic lupus, polyarteritis
      Infectious: **mononucleosis**, hepatitis, Lyme disease, **AIDS**, syphilis,
      Guillain-Barre', leprosy
Familial diseases
      Charcot-Marie-Tooth
      Friedreich's ataxia, and other spinocerebellar degenerations
      Metachromatic leukodystrophy

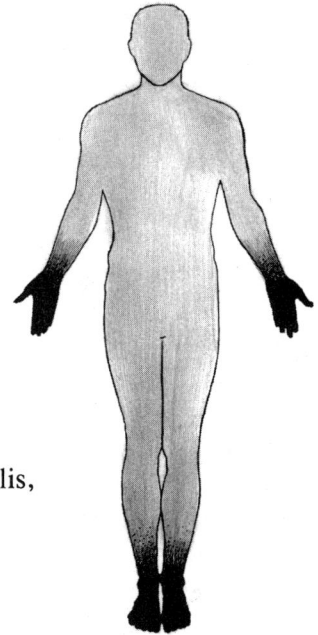

INDICATIONS FOR CT SCAN IN PSYCHIATRIC PATIENTS

•Change in personality or first mental breakdown after age 50
•EEG abnormal
•History of head trauma, alcohol abuse or seizures
•First episode of psychosis
•Focal neurologic findings, cognitive deficits
•Movement disorder
•Resistant eating disorder
•Catatonia
•Dementia or delirium

MRI can be done if the CT scan is abnormal but not conclusive. If the CT scan is normal, MRI can be done if the index of suspicion is high that disease is present. CT is superior in catching calcified brain lesions (Fahr's disease). MRI has better resolution focus and detects multiple sclerosis.

INDICATIONS FOR LUMBAR PUNCTURE
(SPINAL TAP)

Usually indicated if signs of **meningitis** are present: headache, fever, neck rigidity, or subarachnoid **hemorrhage**: (sudden development of worst headache in patients life). **AIDS** patients may have cryptococcal or tuberculous meningitis. In children with **SSPE** who become demented, antimeasles antibody is present in the CSF.

CANCER IN BRAIN

Symptoms include **headache, vomiting, papilledema,** and **neurologic findings**.
50% have mental symptoms. 80% of these are in the frontal or limbic area. Delirium can mean rapid cancerous growth. Incontinence suggests a frontal lobe mass. Deficits of intellect, language, memory loss (recent), and consciousness. Lab: **EEG.** skull x-ray, **CT, MRI,** angiogram.

BRAIN TUMOR-PRIMARY
Gliomas are most common in the 40-50 year age group. Cerebellar tumors disturb coordination and most often are in children.

AIDS: See page 100
May present with primary cerebral lymphoma, or metastasis. Cerebral toxoplasmosis which also occurs in AIDS, is difficult to distinguish symptomatically, with CT, MRI or serology. Cryptococcal meningitis is similar, but has a cryptococcal antigen test that is 95% positive.

METASTATIC CANCER
Usually from the lungs (get x-ray), other sites of origin are the breast, kidney and gastrointestinal tract. Colon cancer is second only to lung cancer as the most common cancer. Symptoms may include blood in feces (hemoccult positive stool), anemia, weight loss or obstructive constipation. The rectal exam may detect this. Breast cancer is the most common for women. Meningeal cancer can occur from the breast, lymphoma, or leukemia. CSF can be checked, but herniation can occur if pressure is high.

SPINAL CANCER
Pain in back, or diffusely in an extremity. Primary tumors may not be cancerous. Metastatic cancer is usually from the prostate [prostate-specific antigen elevated in 98%], breast, lung and kidney.

Distant Effects of cancer in the body includes encephalopathy [diffuse EEG slowing] and immune suppression with brain infection or abscess.

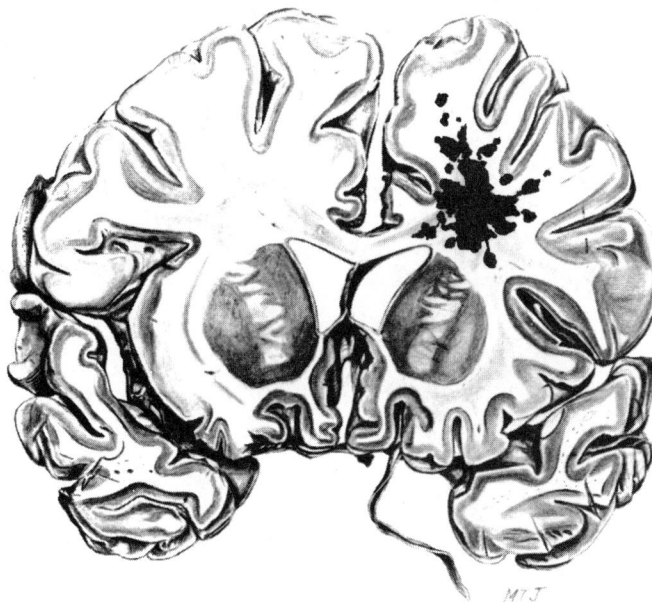

ALZHEIMER'S
50-60% of dementia has this progressive wasting of brain (frontal, temporal) areas. Memory, then language disturbance and personality change occur with loss of neurons in the "substantia innominata" of the brain. At age 65 and 85, 5% and 25% have this. They can be angry, disoriented, and survive usually 8 years, but up to 20.

FAHR'S DISEASE
Calcification of basal ganglia, causing Parkinson's symptoms, psychosis, dementia.

HUNTINGTON'S CHOREA
Is autosomal dominant and has abnormalities in the basal ganglia and caudate nucleus (small), in teenagers, rigid muscles and seizures occur. Irritability and dementia symptoms can start before the continuous rapid lurching, writhing movements begin. Death is usually within 15 years. [CT, MRI, PET scan].

PARKINSON'S DISEASE
Loss of dopamine in the substantia nigra of the brain. Usually occurs in late life, and causes tremor, rigidity, slowed movements, short steps, a mask-like expression, and weakness. Antipsychotic medication blocks dopamine and can cause Parkinson-like symptoms.

PICK'S DISEASE
Similar to Alzheimer's, but rare, and wasting is more confined to frontal and anterior temporal lobes. Death occurs in 2-10 years. "Pick bodies" are found in neurons on autopsy. Language impairment is prominent. Unlike Alzheimer's, visuospacial abilities are preserved, and memory loss occurs later.

WILSON'S DISEASE
Copper deposition causes hepatitis-like picture, corneal ring (green-brown), tremor, slow muscle spasms (dystonia), constant writhing movements (chorea), speech incoordination, psychosis and dementia. Autosomal recessive genetics. The basal ganglia are effected. [serum ceruloplasm low, 24 hour urine copper high, lower alkaline phosphatase]. 1 per 100,000.

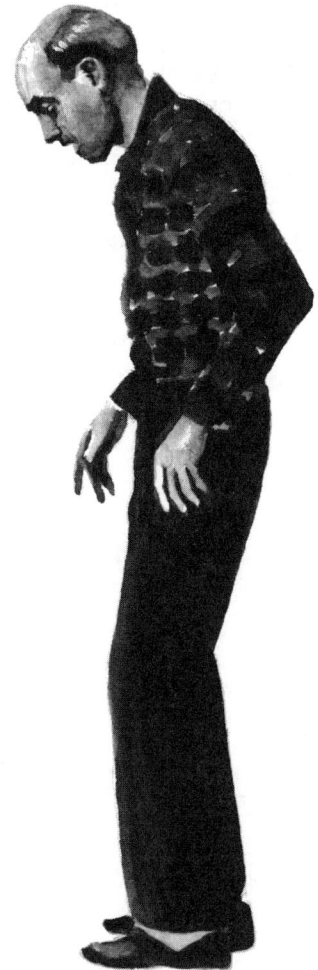

Parkinson's shuffling walk and rigidity

PITUITARY

CUSHING'S DISEASE:
Hyperadrenal signs (page 99) due to overproduction of ACTH by the pituitary.

> Lab blood results are the same as for hyperadrenalism except <u>ACTH is</u> <u>elevated</u>. MRI of pituitary shows adenoma in 50%.

ACROMEGALY:
Excessive growth of hands, feet, jaw. Headaches, visual field loss and personality change, loss of initiative can occur.

> <u>High serum growth hormone</u>. Frequently high fasting prolactin, IGF-1, glucose, liver functions, BUN and serum inorganic phosphorus. MRI shows a pituitary tumor in 90%. Hypothyroid labs can occur.

PANHYPOPITUITARISM:
Mimics anorexia nervosa. Low blood pressure, infertility, depression, loss of sex drive.

> Hypothyroidism, low blood sugar.

THYROID: Both disorders can have anxiety, depression or psychosis. Labs: page 111.

HYPOTHYROIDISM:
Weight gain, fatigue, cold intolerance, constipation, aches, hair loss, brittle nails, dry skin.

> Free T4, FTI are low or borderline low, and/or TSH is high or borderline high (but low if pituitary diseased). Antithyroglobulin or antimitochondrial antibodies may be high.

HYPERTHYROIDISM
Weight loss, High **energy**/pressure, fatigue, heat intolerance, Diarrhea, **palpitations**, sweating.

> Free T4, FTI are high or borderline high, and/or TSH is low or borderline low. Antithyroglobulin or antimitochondrial antibodies may be high.

PARATHYROID

HYPOPARATHYROID

The fall in calcium leads to muscle cramps, tetany, seizure, lethargy, cataracts, retardation, dementia, psychosis, or depression.

> Serum calcium is low, phosphate is high, Parathyroid hormone level is low. CT or x-ray of skull - basal ganglia calcifications, ECG • prolonged QT •T-wave abnormal.

HYPERPARATHYROID:

Decalcification, pains (joints, bones), hypercalcemic, nausea, vomiting, weakness, renal stones, hypertension, uremia, thirst, peptic ulcer, pancreatitis, or constipation. Personality change, psychosis, lethargy or coma can occur.

> Serum potassium and **calcium** are high, serum **phosphate** is low. Urine calcium and phosphate are high. Alkaline phosphatase, uric acid, chloride may increase. **Parathyroid hormone** is high. [Bone cancer and vitamin D intoxication can also raise calcium].

PANCREAS (Low Insulin)

DIABETIC HYPERGLYCEMIA

Drinking much fluid, urinating voluminously, candidal vaginitis in women, weakness, lethargy, delirium, acetone breath.

> Fasting blood sugar is 140 mg/dl or more, glucose tolerance test is abnormal at 1, 2 hours.

(Excess insulin)

HYPOGLYCEMIA: Anxiety, headache, fatigue, sweating.

> Fasting blood sugar is below 65 mg/ml in vulnerable patients

INSULIN OVERDOSE:

Anxiety, psychosis, delirium, coma.

> Glucose levels are between 30-40 mg/ml, severe is below 10mg/ml.

INSULINOMA (85% benign)

Anxiety, psychosis.

> Very low fasting (up to 72 hours in men and up to 24 hours in women), blood sugar, insulin level is not suppressed by low glucose level.

CARCINOMA (Many tumors)

Epigastric discomfort, or pain, weight loss, severe depression, insomnia, jaundice, associated perhaps with diabetes, or alcoholism.

> Pancreatic ultrasound, abdominal cat scan, MRI, biopsy.

ADRENAL

HYPOADRENALISM: (Addison's disease)

Autoimmune or tuberculosis destruction of the surface of the adrenal gland causing deficiency of aldosterone and cortisol. Weakness, abdominal pain, fever, weight loss, nausea, vomiting, low blood pressure, skin pigmentation (diffuse tanning, freckles, darkening), muscle and joint aches, depression, apathy, lethargy, insomnia, psychosis and erratic functioning.

> Serum **potassium**, **BUN**, and perhaps calcium are high, **sodium** and perhaps glucose are low, ACTH given IM does not elevate serum cortisol. If chronic - 8AM **serum cortisol is low** and ACTH is high. Anemia is mild [neutropenia, eosinophilia, lymphocytosis].

HYPERADRENALISM: (Cushing's syndrome)

Central obesity, "moon face", "buffalo hump" shoulders, hypertension, kidney stones, diabetes, bruisability, weakness, and in women menstrual irregularities with hair growth on body. Osteoporosis also occurs. Depression, euphoria, anxiety, psychosis.

> **High serum cortisol** and high free urinary cortisol, resistant to suppression by dexamethasone. **ACTH is low**. High blood and urine glucose, leukocytosis, lymphocytopenia, potassium is low. CT scan of adrenal usually shows a tumor.

PHEOCHROMOCYTOMA:

Attacks of panic, headache, palpitations, hypertension, nausea, chest or abdominal pain, panic, temporary psychosis can occur.

> Elevated 24 hour urinary catacholamines, metanephrines or VMA with creatinine detects most; dietary restrictions apply to make collection. Epinephrine / norepinephrine assay in blood and urine can be done during or after an attack. MRI and CT can help locate tumors. Thyroid tests normal.

TESTICULAR

KLINEFELTERS

1 in 400 males has faulty development of the testes (small) due to XXY genetics, or injury in that area. Breasts are enlarged, penis may be small, and infertility is present. Sex drive is low. Emotional instability and low IQ are typical.

> "Buccal smear" scraping from inner cheek

AIDS

Wasting, weight loss, diarrhea, fatigue, fevers, night sweats and lymph node disease due to HIV infection. AIDS has opportunistic infections (pneumonias cause low oxygen, in brain causes damage), aggressive cancers (kaposi's sarcoma - purple-brown skin patches, brain cancer), and neurologic deterioration (dementia, confusion, nerve disease). [HIV antibody+, T_4 cell count declines]. See cancer, page 95.

CREUTZFELDT-JACOB DISEASE

Can be in adults in their 50's, and kills in 1 year. Muscle twitches / jerks, incoordination of walkingand speech, writhing in hands, dementia, and sleepiness occur. Transmission is medical (corneal transplants, intracerebral electrodes, biopsy) [EEG period complexes]

CYTOMEGALOVIRUS

Malaise, muscle and joint aches, no sore throat (unlike mononucleosis). [Abnormal liver function tests, atypical lymphocytes, CMV (IgM, IgG) +].

EBSTEIN-BARR VIRUS - (MONONUCLEOSIS)

Fever, sore throat, enlarged lymphnoids, rash, nausea, headache, hepatitis, myocarditis and even encephalitis can occur. Fatigue, depression, anxiety and panic are common. [EBV-IgM is high acutely, then IgG is high in 3 weeks, granulocytopenia followed within 1 week by lymphocytic leukocytosis].

HEPATITIS

Severe anorexia, malaise, muscle and joint aches, fatigue, upper respiratory symptoms, fever, mild upper right adominal pain, jaundice within 10 days. [elevated liver enzymes: ALT]

Hepatitis A
From contaminated water or food, may persist for a year [anti-HAV].

Hepatitis B
From infected blood or body secretions (IV drug abuse, sexual contact, accidental needle stick), 10% develop chronic liver disease [HBsAg - hepatitis B surface antigen].

Hepatitis D
May co-infect with hepatitis B [Anti-HDV].

Hepatitis C
Similar to hepatitis B, but greater than 50% develop chronic hepatitis. 80% of post transfusion hepatitis is due to this. 40% of cases are due to IV drug abuse [Anti-HCV].

HERPES SIMPLEX

Can cause the most common focal encephalitis [temporal lobe seizure foci on EEG, "mass-like" lesion on scans]. Symptoms can include loss of smell, hallucinations (smell and taste), memory loss, and personality changes. Bleeding tissue breakdown can cause fever, headache, seizures, fatigue and coma. Vicious cycle of stress and brain inflammation. [SPECT imaging may identify herpes encephalitis].

LYME DISEASE

A tick bite can cause rash. Fatigue, headache, spasticity, staggering and dementia-like symptoms can occur years after the bite and rash. Serology turns positive late. False positives can occur from syphilis, mononucleosis and autoimmune disorders. [serum antibodies to Borrelia burgdorferi]

NEUROSYPHILIS

"General paresis" appears in 10-15 years in 15% of those who had a primary syphilis infection. Abnormal sensations, shooting pains, and dementia occur. "Gumma" lesions cause muscle and bone pains as well as breathing difficulties. Heart lesions can be life threatening. Incidence is increasing with AIDS. [VDRL / RPR, treponema antibody test (FTA-ABS, MHA-TP), CSF-VDRL]

MULTIPLE SCLEROSIS
Most common neurologic illness of young adults. Episodic sensory deteriorations, emotionality, optic neuritis (blindness) can occur, incontinence, unsteady gait and voice. Frequency is 1 per 1,000-2,000 people. [MRI shows scattered demyelination, CSF-possible high gamma globulin].

MYASTHENIA GRAVIS
Antibodies bind acetylcholine receptors causing loss of muscle strength with quick fatigue. Symptoms may include double vision, difficulty swallowing and weakness with activity.

[Diagnosis is with Edrophonium 2 mg., 8 mg.]

POLYARTERITIS NODOSA
Destructive inflammation of blood vessels causing organ infarctions and joint-muscle pain, fever, hypertension, abdominal pain, nausea and vomiting.

[Sedimentation rate high, protein and blood in urine, anemia, elevated WBC count, biopsy.]

RHEUMATIC FEVER
A streptococcal immune process can cause fatigue, mental symptoms, delirium, carditis, arthritis, rash, or uncontrollable movements (chorea-3%). A recent sore throat is in 20%.

[ASLO titer, throat culture, high WBC's, high ESR, C-reactive protein present, prolonged PR on ECG]

SSPE (Subacute sclerosing panencephalitis)
In childhood, usually following measles infection or vaccination, characterized by demyelination, misbehavior, muscle jerks (myoclonus), seizures

[CSF measles antibodies elevated initially, EEG - periodic complexes]

SYSTEMIC LUPUS ERYTHEMATOSIS (1 in 33,000)
Autoimmune disorder effecting usually young women with joint aches (90%) and sunlight rashes. Kidney disease, seizures and anemia can occur. Anxiety, depression, psychosis, delirium or dementia are possible.

[Positive antinuclear antibody (ANA) with high titer of native DNA. LE prep and antibody to Sm can be positive]

TEMPORAL ARTERITIS
One sided headache, fever, cough, a painful shoulder or pelvis and shoulder girdle. Onset is abrupt.

[Often has anemia and a high sedimentation rate.]

HYPONATREMIA
Too much antidiuretic hormone causes excess water reabsorption and possibly delusional depression.

[Low Sodium]

KIDNEY FAILURE / ENCEPHALOPATHY
Can cause anything from anxiety to dementia. They may experience nausea, itching and persistent hiccups. A restless legs syndrome, burning feet and twitching are due to sensorimotor neuropathy.

[BUN and creatinine high, urine output low, nerve conduction velocities effected].

LIVER FAILURE / ENCEPHALOPATHY
Can cause psychosis, depression, drowsiness and coma. Nausea, asterixis (hand flapping), spiderlike blood vessels on skin, palms flushed, reflexes increased, liver enlarged or small, jaundice is late.

[liver functions abnormal, EEG slowing, serum ammonia high].

PORPHYRIA (Acute intermittent)
Autosomal dominant defect causing intermittent abdominal pain (nausea, vomiting), psychosis, seizures, and/or neuropathy (visual loss, paralysis of all 4 limbs and of breathing is possible). It is precipitated by alcohol, barbiturates, menstruation, pregnancy, a variety of medications, infection or starvation.

[High urine porphobilinogen and aminolevulinic acid, low sodium often, especially during attacks].

SEIZURE DISORDERS
The most common (1%) chronic neurologic disease. Electrical instability can be partial, contained, yet symptomatic. Generalized epilepsy with unconsciousness is more common. 30% are hereditary.

[EEG is positive in 40%, repeated testing identifies 90%. MRI rules out structural lesions. Also indicated are serum electrolytes, calcium, magnesium, CBC, and a urine drug screen (cocaine / amphetamine intoxication, alcohol / benzodiazepine withdrawl). Lumbar puncture can help for trauma, meningitis, encephalitis. Kidney, liver and cardiopulmonary status (blood gases) can be checked. Toxins such as lead, mercury and carbon monoxide cause seizures. Thyrotoxicosis and porphyria can also.]

TOXIC METAL (HEAVY)

Lead: Colicky pain, constipation, headache, irritability, learning disability, wrist drop.

Mercury: Contaminated fish or fungicides on seeds have caused confusion, psychosis, headache, fatigue, staggering, tremors, seizures and birth defects. Mercury vaporizes at room temperature and can be inhaled by workers in the electrochemical industry.

Manganese: Can cause psychosis and a Parkinson-like syndrome.

Aluminum: Causes dementia.

Arsenic: Fatigue, blackouts, hair loss, thick palms and soles, anemia.

TRAUMATIC

HEAD TRAUMA:
Can cause headache, dizziness, loss of consciousness, skull fracture ("racoon eyes", blood from ear canal) [x-ray], brain fluid [CSF] from nose or ears [glucose+], cranial nerve paralysis (1,2,3,4,5,7,8), intracranial hemorrhage or edema [CT scan], neck trauma (all comatose patients should have lateral cervical x-rays), normal pressure hydrocephalus [CT/MRI, cisternography], focal injury, inflammation and seizures. [EEG]. Victims can have confusion, amnesia (healing stops after a year), distractibility, impulsivity, aggression or other mental changes.

NORMAL PRESSURE HYDROCEPHALUS:
Head injury, intracranial bleeding or inflammation can cause excess spinal fluid to dilate ventricles. Symptoms include gait incoordination, incontinence and dementia. [CT/MRI, cisternography, CSF withdrawal]

VITAMIN DEFICIENCY / MALABSORPTION

Thiamine Deficiency: (Beriberi means "I cannot do anything") is a factor in alcoholism causing neuritis, reversible Wernicke's (confusion, gait incoordination, eye paralysis) - and often irreversible Korsakoff's (inability to form new memories or remember old ones). A polished rice diet can also cause this. Cardiac pathology and swelling can occur.

Cobalamin (B_{12}) Deficiency: Is usually due to an autoimmune based failure of stomach cells to secrete intrinsic factor necessary for absorption of B_{12} from the intestine. Neurologic changes (depression, psychosis, dementia) may precede the "pernicious anemia" [CBC may show macrocytic, megaloblastic anemia]. [serum B_{12} low, or B_{12} bioactivity assay low, schilling test "+"].

Niacin Deficiency (Pellagra): May occur with alcoholism, vegetarian or corn diets, starvation, and genetically. Symptoms may include anorexia, sore inflamed mouth and tongue, **D**iarrhea, **D**ermatitis (dark scaling skin) on sunlit and trauma areas, **D**ementia (insomnia, irritability, psychosis, confusion), and **D**eath.

Folate Deficiency: Can cause burning feet, restless legs syndrome and depression, usually in alcoholics, anorexics, and the elderly who do not eat enough fruits and vegetables. [CBC may show a macrocytic anemia and low serum folate]. Pregnancy, malabsorption, dialysis, and dilantin (phenytoin) can also cause deficiency.

Pyridoxine (B_6) Deficiency: May occur from alcoholism, birth control pills or isoniazid. Symptoms can include mouth and tongue soreness, lip fissures, irritability, neuropathy, weakness, anemia and seizures.

Reference for Abnormal Lab Data
(Approximate, not Comprehensive)

Test	Comments
Acid phosphatase	**High** in prostate cancer, prostatic enlargement, platelet destruction, bone disease, and hyperplasia. PSA test is superior and replacing this test.
Adrenocorticotropic hormone (ACTH)	**High** in Cushing's disease, and from stress. May be increased in seizures, psychotic disorders. **High** in Addison's disease. AM samples are two-fold Higher than PM so sampling time is important. **Low** (suppressed) when corticosteroids are being given.
Alanine aminotransferase (ALT) (formerly SGPT)	**High** in hepatitis, cirrhosis, liver metastases. **Low** in vitamin B12 deficiency.
Albumin	**High** in dehydration. **Low** in malnutrition, liver, kidney or severe skin disease, burns, multiple myeloma, cancer.
Aldolase	**High** in ipecac abuse (i.e., bulimic patients), schizophrenia (60-80%), and duchenne's muscular dystrophy.
Alkaline phosphatase	**High** in Paget's disease, hyperparathyroidism, liver disease, liver metastases, heart failure, with phenothiazines use. **Low** in pernicious anemia (vitamin B_{12} deficiency).
Ammonia (serum)	**High** in liver encephalopathy.
Amylase (serum)	Can be increased in bulimia nervosa and pancreatitis.
Antinuclear antibodies (ANA)	Found in 98% of systemic lupus erythematosus (SLE) patients and drug-induced lupus. The ANA panel includes: [**Anti-DNA** has a Higher specificity for SLE and can be used to monitor progress.] [**Plasma complements (C3,C4)** for SLE reveal C3a and C5a activation products suggestive of CNS lupus].
Aspartate aminotransferase (AST) (formerly SGOT)	**High** in heart attack, liver disease, pancreatitis, eclampsia, brain damage, alcoholism. **Low** in vitamin B_6 deficiency, terminal stages of liver damage.
Bicarbonate (serum)	**Low** with hyperventilation (panic disorder), anabolic steroid abuse. Can be elevated in patients with bulimia nervosa, laxative abuse, vomiting.

Test	Comments
Bilirubin	**Increased** in cholestatic liver disease, hemolysis or by genetics. Jaundice can result.
Blood urea nitrogen (BUN)	**Elevated** in kidney disease, dehydration and is associated with lethargy, delirium. Can increase toxic potential of lithium.
Borrelia burgdorferi, serum antibodies	Lyme disease, see page 100.
Bromide (serum)	Bromide can cause psychosis, delirium, dementia, and as sleep medicines have been discontinued. Serum chloride may be elevated.
Brucellosis (agglutinin test)	Depression, fatigue and anxiety in people working with domestic animals (farmers, vets, meatpackers).
Caffeine level (serum)	For suspected caffeinism.
Calcium (Ca), (serum)	Low or high with renal failure. **High** due to cancer of all types (especially metastatic), hyperparathyroidism (very high levels occur in parathyroid cancer), lab error-excess tourniquet time (repeat), Addison's, hyperthyroidism, cancer (parathyroid hormone low), bone fracture, immobilization, acute illness, familial (urine calcium low), antacids (sodium bicarbonate, calcium carbonate), thiazide diuretics, tuberculosis, histoplasmosis, coccidiomycosis, leprosy, foreign body granuloma. **Low** calcium due to hypoparathyroidism, malabsorption (calcium, magnesium, vitamin D), diuretics (loop), phenytoin, rapid transfusion, acute pancreatitis, parathyroid removal, metastatic cancer (breast, prostate especially), chemotherapy (phosphates), infants fed cow's milk.
Carotid Ultrasound	To check for ischemia, atherosclerosis and occlusive disease.
Catecholamines (urinary screen and 24 hour)	**High** in pheochromocytoma. Yet stress, alcohol, decongestants, MAOI, lithium, benzodiazepines, phenothiazines, bananas, citrus, vanilla, tea, coffee, chocolate, and other things can increase levels. Dietary restrictions during the test are important.
Cerebrospinal fluid (CSF)	Increase WBC count and protein, with decreased glucose in infection (bacterial, viral, TB and fungal meningitis). VDRL"+" in 60% of neurosyphilis cases. Bloody in subarachnoid hemorrhage.
Ceruloplasmin (serum) Copper (24 hour urine)	**Low** in Wilson's disease. **High** in Wilson's disease.

Test	Comments
Chloride (Cl) (serum)	**Low** in patients with vomiting, diuretic therapy, or kidney disease. Mild **elevation** in hyperventilation syndrome, excess mineral intake or dehydration.
Cholesterol, triglycerides	50% of Americans have cholesterol above 200 causing atherosclerotic heart disease (Reference 8). Too much meat, and not enough vegetables and fiber is usual cause. [A lipid profile differentiates healthy HDL from unhealthy LDL levels.]
Coombs' test, direct and indirect	Evaluation of drug-induced hemolytic anemias, such as those secondary to chlorpromazine (thorazine), or phenytoin (dilantin).
Cortisol, serum	Cortisol (hydrocortisone) highest on waking, lowest at bedtime. Cortisol increases with exercise, trauma, infection and other stresses. It dampens dangerous overactivity of the body's defenses. An elevated level may indicate Cushing's disease or syndrome. **High** - Adrenal hyperplasia or adenoma (Cushing's), pregnancy, depression, stress. **Low** - Adrenogenital syndrome, adrenocorticoinsufficiency (Addison's). Use dexamethasone suppression test to rule out Cushing's.
Creatine phosphokinase (CPK)	**High** in neuroleptic malignant syndrome, intramuscular injection, with restraints, dystonic reactions; rhabdomyolysis (secondary to substance abuse) or Duchenne's muscular dystrophy. Asymptomatic elevations occur with antipsychotics.
Creatinine, serum	**Elevated** in kidney disease.
Doppler ultrasound	Used for Carotid occlusion, low penile blood flow in impotence, thyroid and parathyroid adenomas.
Drug testing	See page 121
Echocardiogram	10-40% of patients with panic disorder have mitral valve prolapse.
Electroencephalogram (EEG)	Seizures, brain lesions, shortened REM latency occurs in depression. **Stupor**: High-voltage activity. **Excitement:** Low-voltage fast activity. Nonorganic cases (dissociative disorders): alpha activity which responds to auditory and visual stimuli is present in background. Periodic high voltage, slow wave complexes occur in Creutzfeldt-Jacob disease.

106

Test	Comments
Epstein- Barr virus (EBV); cytomegalovirus (CMV) (IgG, IgM)	Either may present with fatigue, depression, mood changes, or anxiety. EBV is mononucleosis. The IgM fraction indicates acute, ongoing infection. A chronic mononucleosis may exist.
Erythrocyte sedimentation rate (ESR)	A **high** ESR results from infectious, inflammatory, autoimmune, or malignant disease. This test is mainly useful for monitoring temporal arteritis and polymyalgia rheumatica. A high ESR is usually followed with a repeat test in several months, rather than exhaustively searching for disease.
Estrogen	**Low** in menopausal depression and sometimes premenstrual syndrome. Menopause has low estradiol (5-25 pg/ml) elevated LH (30-105 m1U/m1) and FSH (40-250 m1U/ml).
Ferritin, serum	Most sensitive test for low iron.
Folate (folic acid) serum	Usually checked with serum B_{12} level and may be low with alcohol dependence, use of phenytoin (dilantin), oral contraceptives, estrogen, pregnancy, dialysis or skin exfoliation.
Follicle-stimulating hormone (FSH)	**High** in postmenopausal women; **low** in patients with panhypopituitarism, high normal in starvation
Glucose, fasting blood sugar (FBS)	**Low** in hyperinsulinism (subcutaneous injections or tumor), functional hypoglycemia due to vagas parasympathetic overactivity (anxiety, irritability, headache, hunger), alcohol induced, and normal variation. Also obvious failure of the pituitary, thyroid, adrenal, liver, or kidney can do this. **High** in diabetes, acromegaly, Cushing's syndrome, pheochromocytoma, medications (sympathomimetic drugs, steroids, niacin, thiazide diuretics, phenytoin), liver disease and pancreatitis.
Glutamyl transaminase, serum	**High** in alcohol abuse, cirrhosis, liver disease, biliary obstruction.
Hematocrit (Hct); hemoglobin (Hb)	MCV is **low** in iron deficiency anemia and anemia of chronic disease; MCV is increased in (megaloblastic) B_{12} or folate deficiency anemia, in liver disease, and hypothyroid anemia.
Hepatitis	See page 100.
Holter monitor	Evaluation of panic with palpitations or other heart symptoms.
Human immunodeficiency virus (HIV) [HIV antibody test]	For AIDS dementia, personality change, depression or psychosis. See page 95, 100.

Test	Comments
17-Hydroxycorticosteriod	**High** in hyperadrenocorticalism, depression, alcoholism, and steroid abuse.
Iron, serum	Anemia due to iron deficiency. Use TIBC (% saturation) and iron for differential diagnosis of anemias.
Lactate dehydrogenase (LDH)	LDH is found in nearly all tissues, but primarily in the heart, kidney, liver, muscles, and RBCs. Thus heart attack, kidney or liver disease, seizures, brain damage, pulmonary infarction, megaloblastic anemia, and even rough handling of the blood specimen tube can elevate this. Isoenzyme for LDH can help identify which system is effected.
Lipid profile	Checks total cholesterol, HDL (good cholesterol), LDL (bad cholesterol) and triglycerides.
Lupus anticoagulant (LA)	In a test tube, this can be positive in patients taking phenothiazines (thorazine), or with cancer or auto-immune conditions such as SLE, as well as in normal individuals. In the body, thrombosis risk is increased.
Lupus erythematosus (LE) test	Positive in systemic lupus erythematosus (SLE) but many drugs can cause a false positive result (phenothiazines, barbiturates, phenytoin, procainamide). [ANA, antiDNA, and C_3/C_4 can also be checked]. A lupus panel exists, but does not include C_3/C_4. See ANA.
Luteinizing hormone (LH)	**Increased** in ovarian failure, or menopausal lack of menses. **Decreased** in pituitary failure lack of menses, estrogen or testosterone administration, or an estrogen/progesterone producing tumor (ovary, adrenal). Opioid abuse also lowers LH.
Magnesium, serum	**Low** magnesium symptoms include agitation, delirium, and seizures. Low levels occur in up to 60% of critically ill hospitalized patients, alcoholics, the malnourished, patients with chronic diarrhea, diabetic ketoacidosis, diuretic treatment, High calcium, hyperparathyroidism, vitamin D therapy, with certain antibiotics. **Low** calcium and low potassium are often present. **High** magnesium occurs in kidney failure.
MCV (mean corpuscular volume) (average volume of a red blood cell)	See Hct / Hb
Metal (heavy) intoxication (serum or urinary)	Lead, mercury, manganese, aluminum, arsenic
Myoglobin, urine	**High** in neuroleptic malignant syndrome; in PCP or cocaine intoxication and in patients in restraints.

Test	Comments
Nocturnal penile tumescence	Erections associated with rapid eye movement (REM) sleep differentiate organic from functional causes of impotence.
Parathyroid (parathormone) hormone	**Low** level causes low calcium-hypoparathyroidism. **High** level causes high calcium-hyperparathyroidism. See page 98.
Phosphorus, serum	**Decreased** in alcoholism, starvation, malabsorption, hyperventilation, diabetes mellitis, hyperparathyroidism, High calcium, hyperthyroidism, kidney defects, glucose, steroids, estrogen, oral contraceptives, aspirin poisoning, severe burns, low magnesium, low potassium, vitamin D deficiency. **Increased** in hypoparathyroidism, low calcium, acromegaly, kidney failure, stress or injury, rhabdomyolysis, chemotherapy, laxatives or enemas with phosphate, vitamin D excess.
Platelet count	**Lowered** by some psychotropic medications (carbamazepine, clozapine, phenothiazines), and leukemias
Porphobilinogen (PBG) 24 hour urine collection or fresh random sample	**High** in acute porphyria. See page 102.
Potassium (K), serum	**Low** levels cause weakness, fatigue, constipation, and muscle cramps. Low potassium is most frequently due to diuretics, laxative abuse, vomiting, cirrhosis, Cushing's, Conn's, familial, metabolic alkalosis. **High** levels cause weakness, bloating, and diarrhea. Slowed heart rate, ventricular fibrillation and cardiac arrest can occur. High potassium may be due to collection technique (delayed separation of serum from clot, fist clenching during collection), severe dehydration, kidney failure, exercise, burns, physical injury, metabolic acidosis, low insulin, familial ("periodic paralysis"), medications, potassium supplementation.
Prolactin, serum	Prolactin inhibitory factor is dopamine; Prolactin is **increased** by antipsychotic treatment, cocaine withdrawl, seizures, pregnancy, lactation, estrogen therapy, hypothyroidism, or advanced renal insufficiency. A pituitary adenoma can also increase prolactin. This causes lactation and menstrual disturbances in women, but in men, low libido, erection problems and infertility. Prolactin is **decreased** in panhypopituitarism, and L-Dopa or ergot alkaloid treatment.
Pregnancy [HCG test]	Blood test can be positive at or just before the expected menses. The urine test can be positive 2 weeks after conception. HCG is human chorionic ganadotropin hormone.

Test	Comments
Prostate specific antigin (PSA)	**High** in prostate cancer; good screening test.
Protein, total serum	**High** in multiple myloma, hypothyroidism, inflammation, lupus, arthritis, cancer, obstructive jaundice, diabetes, nephrotic syndrome, iron deficiency or low albumin. **Low** in liver disease, starvation, overhydration, or emphysema. Protein bound medicines (not lithium) show more activity.
Prothrombin time (PT)	**Elevated** in liver disease and patients with lupus anticoagulant.
Reticulocyte count (red blood cell production in bone marrow)	**Low** when suppressed by carbamazepine, or in marrow aplasia or replacement due to leukemic cells. **High** in hemolysis, acute blood loss and in response to replacement of a deficiency (iron, B_{12}, folate).
Salicylate, serum	Toxic levels cause nausea, stomach inflammation, rapid breathing and heart rate, ringing in the ears, confusion, psychosis, seizures, coma, fever, cardiovascular collapse and death. PTT is usually elevated.
Sodium (NA), serum	**Low** due to hyperglycemia, fluid depletion or overload (heart failure, cirrhosis, nephrotic syndrome), water intoxication, inappropriate ADH secretion (lithium,carbamazepine), postoperative, hypothyroidism, chronic beer excess (cirrhosis), diuretics, diarrhea, AIDS, steroids. **High** due to excessive salt intake, sweating, stool water loss, diabetes (glycosuria diuresis).
Syphilis	The VDRL test for syphilis may be low or normal in late forms of syphilis (neurosyphilis), but positive in primary or secondary forms. A false positive VDRL can occur from SLE, rheumatoid arthritis, IV drug abuse and mononucleosis as well as some other infectious diseases. The RPR is the most common screening test for syphilis. The <u>FTA-ABS</u> (florescent treponemal antibody test) is sensitive particularly for late stage syphilis. Lupus or lyme disease can cause false positive results with FTA-ABS. Positive VDRL's or RPR's should be confirmed with the FTA-ABS.

Test	Comments
Testosterone, serum	**High** in anabolic steroid abuse. **Low** with low sex drive. Low with medroxyprogesterone treatment of sex offenders.
Thyroid function tests	* **Serum free T4** is **elevated** in hyperthyroidism and **decreased** in hypothyroidism. It is also decreased in nonthyroidal illness such as with alcoholic liver disease, malnutrition, poorly controlled diabetes, chronic renal failure, acute myocardial infarction, major surgery, trauma, leukemia, birth trauma, prematurity, and low oxygen. Monitoring the reduction of T4 by anti-thyroid drugs is useful to gauge treatment effectiveness. **Serum Total T4** normally follows the TBG concentration and binding capacity. **TBG** (thyroid binding globulin) is elevated by estrogen (oral contraceptives), pregnancy, in the newborn, with methadone, heroin, perphenazine (trilafon), porphyria, liver inflammation, and a hereditary X-linked trait. Total T4 and T3 are also increased, but Free T4 should be normal. **TBG** is reduced by androgens, steroids, phenytoin (Dilantin), carbamazepine (Tegretal), colestipol with niacin, malnutrition, fasting, severe or chronic illness, cirrhosis, nephrotic syndrome and heredity. TBG capacity is lowered when drugs occupy binding sites (aspirin, dilantin, furosamide). Total T4 and T3 are reduced, but Free T4 should be normal. **T3RU** (T3 resin uptake) is elevated in hyperthyroidism and protein depletion states (malnutrition, liver disease, nephrotic syndrome), and is decreased in hypothyroidism, and with increased protein (pregnancy, oral contraceptive, estrogen). * **Free thyroxine index (FTI)** is for general screening of thyroid function. It is the serum total T4 multiplied by the T3 resin uptake (T3RU) and a factor. **Serum Total T3** - When other tests are borderline, this can detect T3 - toxicosis to confirm hyperthyroidism. There exists nonthyroidal illness where T3 is low. * **Low TSH** - **less than 0.1** microunit/ml is hyperthyroidism. - **less than 0.5** is "subclinical" hyperthyroidism. [Yet TSH can be lowered by cigarette smoking, old age, kidney failure, Cushing's syndrome or other severe illnesses. Medicines can suppress TSH: **thyroid medicines**, dopamine, glucocorticoids, endorphines, somatostatin. Hypothalamic malfunction (low TRH) can decrease TSH.] -TSH is not a reliable index to judge effectiveness of treatment, but is good to gauge maximum dose a post menopausal female can have without causing **demineralization**. TSH can stay suppressed for months after the thyroid is normalized.

Test	Comments
Thryoid (continued)	**High TSH** - **Greater than 5** microunits/ml may indicate "subclinical" or impending hypothyroidism. - **Greater than 10** indicates hypothyroidism. In this situation, **TSH is useful to monitor treatment effectiveness**. [TSH elevates with hypothyroidism but also due to cancer in the pituitary, or pituitary resistance to negative feedback by thyroid]. 2% of the elderly have a normal, mild elevation of TSH. 14% of psychiatric admissions show a transcient elevation of TSH that usually returns to normal [Reference 5]. **Circulating thyroid antibodies** help to identify autoimmune thyroid disease. This includes **antithyroglobulin antibody, anti-mitochondrial antibody,** antithyroid peroxidase (anti-TPO) antibody, thyroid stimulating antibody, thyroid stimulating blocking antibody. **Thyroid Scan** - Differentiates different types of hyperthyroidism and determines the likelihood of cancer. Fine-needle aspiration differentiates thyroid nodules as non-cancerous versus cancerous. Ultrasound differentiates cystic from solid thyroid nodules. MRI and CT scan also are helpful.
Urinalysis	Can be used for drug screening (see page 121), prelithium workup and organicity workup.
Urinary creatinine	**High** in kidney failure, dehydration. Checked in pre-treatment workup for lithium.
Vitamin A, serum	Excessive vitamin A causes changes in mental status and increased intracranial pressure.
Vitamin B_{12}, serum	Deficiency causes megaloblastic anemia and dementia and is often associated with chronic alcohol abuse or autoimmune pernicious anemia.
White blood cell (WBC)	Leukopenia and agranulocytosis are associated with some psychotropic medications (phenothiazines, carbamazepine, clozapine). Leukocytosis occurs with lithium and neuroleptic malignant syndrome.

ADDICTION, SUBSTANCE ABUSE

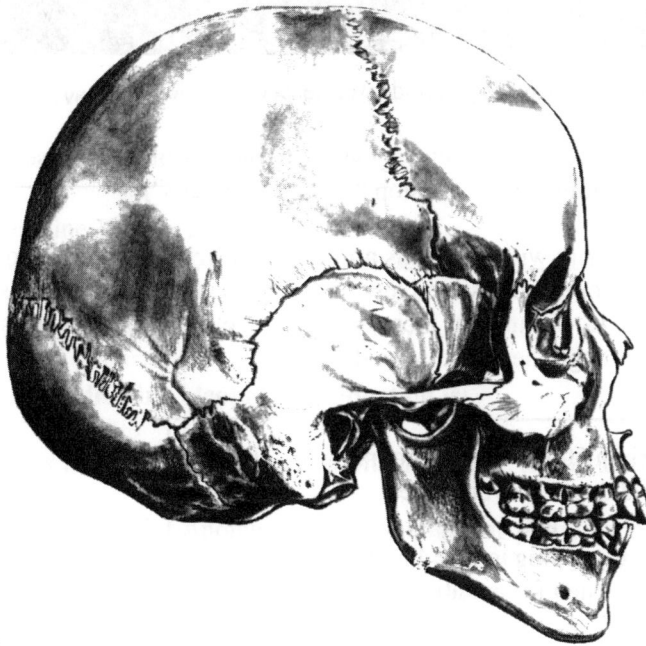

Sedative Hypnotic Addiction (benzodiazepines, for example Valium, barbituates)

Intoxication: Slurring, incoordination, drowsiness, coma, death.

Withdrawal: Sweating, pulse above 100, anxiety, agitation, tremor, insomnia, nausea, vomiting, muscle aches, confusion, hallucinations, seizures, death.

Detoxification is identical, but more prolonged (weeks rather than days) than alcoholism detox. It is also more dangerous: sudden discontinuation of sedative hypnotics (especially for high dose addictions) can cause disorientation, seizures and death. Again, the chemical imbalance should be sought and corrected, during and after detoxification. The 12 step meetings that most closely match the patients personality or preference should be chosen (Alcoholics Anonymous, Narcotics Anonymous, Cocaine Anonymous) regardless of what addiction occurred.

Opiate Addiction (heroin, "tar", Vicodan, Perodan, Dilaudid, codeine, Demerol, etc.)

Intoxication: Pupils constrict, speech slurs, slow heart rate, constipation, weight loss, drowsiness, coma, death.

Withdrawal: Distress, pupils dilate, nausea, vomiting, muscle aches, runny nose, tearing, "goose flesh", sweating, diarrhea, yawning, fever, rapid pulse, high blood pressure, rapid breathing.

This is one of the hardest addictions, next to cocaine to stop, due to relapse. It is also usually a difficult detox, so medications have to be generous for 5 days.

> Clonidine (0.1-0.2mg.) four times daily (as long as systolic blood pressure is greater than 90).
> Robaxin (500mg): 2-3 tablets, four times daily as needed for muscle cramps.
> Bentyl (20mg.) 4 times per day as needed for stomach cramps.
> Librium (50mg.) every 4 hours for moderate sedation, hold doses if oversedated. Librium (50mg.) every 4 hours as needed for agitation.

> Phenobarbitol (30mg), 4 times per day can be added for especially difficult detoxes.

After 5 days, the heavily used librium, and phenobarbitol, then clonidine can start to be tapered.

I believe all opiate addicts are chemically imbalanced, (often in the Protocol 2 or 3 area) and so the protocols are initiated. Note that detoxification medicines are used to maintain comfort during this. If a protocol psychotropic medicine results in more detox medicine requirement within 24-48 hours, it is failing.

116

Tegretal is not narcotic, yet feels like heroin according to many addicts. This has been frequently successful.

Tegretal (100mg.) 2-3 times per day

Lithium also often matches the constitution of these patients.

Eskalith (300mg.) 2-3 times per day

Trexan after the detox prevents euphoria if the patient abuses opiate again. It can remove the incentive of feeling high and help them to stay sober. Yet addicts sometimes stop this to relapse.

Trexan (Naltrexone) (100mg.) 3 times per week.

After hospitalization, the chances for success are increased by:
(1) Completely fixing the underlying chemical imbalance (the person feels right).
(2) Rigorous NA (Narcotics Anonymous) 12 step meeting participation (daily for 90 days initially), and getting a sponsor.
(3) Trexan 3 times per week

Cocaine and Amphetamine Addiction ("crack, crank, ecstacy")

Intoxication: Agitation and hyperactivity, confusion, psychosis, dilated pupils, rapid heart rate, sweating, high blood pressure, chronic hoarseness, nose bleeds, nausea, vomiting, weight loss, weakness, decreased breathing, chest pain, heart irregularity, delirium, seizures, muscle spasms, migraine, strokes, fever, death.

Withdrawl: Agitation, insomnia, then fatigue and excess sleeping, unpleasant dreams, then agitation, depression and eating.

Other addictions have withdrawl syndromes that are characterized by agitation and anxiety. Cocaine and amphetamine addiction are different. After the first detox librium dose in the hospital, sleep may last for a day. As the patient wakes up, intense craving and distress may need medicated.

Librium 25-50mg: every 4 hours as needed for agitation	
Tyrosine 500mg Amantadine 100mg	3 times per day to block craving.

For extreme agitation or violence, antipsychotic can be added:

Haldol 5mg Cogentin 1mg	orally or IM 3 times daily as needed

117

Protocol #1 can be customized to this addiction. Instead of prescribing a serotonin agent, a NE. agent is used since this one decreases cocaine or amphetamine craving over a 2 week period:

```
Norpramine 25mg. in the A.M., raise as tolerated by
25mg. daily, up to an average of 150mg. in A.M. daily.
```

When the patient is comfortable, all the detox medications can be discontinued. The Norpramine can be taken long term.

If worsening occurs with Norpramine, stop it and try the standard protocols (page 40). Drastic destabilization on Norpramine usually is due to underlying manic depression.

```
Antidote: Stelazine 2mg.
```

These patients can be jumpy, agitated, and possibly brain injured. Tegretal is often a favorite because it relaxes them and is compatible with their injury.

```
Tegretal 100mg. 2-3 times a day
```

The formula to maximize chances of success is:

    (1)   Completely fix the chemical imbalance (the person feels good).

    (2)   Rigorous 12 step meeting participation (daily for 90 days initially) and getting a sponsor. Sometimes AA is more useful then CA for these patients because of its stability.

Marijuana Addiction ("pot, weed")

Intoxication: Sleepiness, ECG abnormalities, decreased testosterone levels, or abnormal menstruation.

Withdrawal: Insomnia, nausea, muscle pains, irritability.

I use the Protocols (1-5) to help this. Marijuana may elevate dopamine 6-fold.

Nicotine Addiction (tobacco)

Nicotine (like the opiates, cocaine, alcohol and marijuana) stimulates dopamine in a "reward region" of the brain causing addiction. It enhances alertness, relaxes muscles and is a primary cause of cancer.

Withdrawal: Irritability, anxiety, insomnia, headache, tremor, fatigue and craving, lasting sometimes for months.

Protocols 1-5 can be initiated prior to and during nicotine "detox." Lung cancer is a most preventable and least curable cancer. Prevention is the key.

Nicorette Gum can be used instead of skin patches. There are 96 chewing pieces per box. Patients should read the package insert. First, smoking is stopped.

118

Nicorette DS	:	4mg nicotine / piece - maximum 20 pieces / day	
Nicorette	:	2mg nicotine / piece - maximum 30 pieces / day	
Cigarettes (USA)	:	11mg nicotine each	

Patients should start with a 2 or 4 mg piece, and learn to chew slowly (30 minutes per piece), and on a fixed schedule (every 1-2 hours). Weaning should be started in 2-3 months, and completed by 4-6 months.

NICOTINE WITHDRAWAL SKIN PATCH SYSTEMS

(1)   Patients must stop smoking immediately prior to and during usage of the nicotine skin patches. They should read the instructions that come with the medicine.

(2)   Skin patches are replaced once daily to different skin areas that are non-hairy, dry and clean, and on the upper body or upper outer arms.

(3)   Skin sites should not be reused for a week.

	Patch Duration	Dosing Withdrawal Schedule	Doses For: • Heart Disease • Wt. below 100 lbs • Smoking less than 10 cigarettes per day
Habitrol	24hrs. #30/box	21mg: 6 wks, then 14mg: 2 wks, then 7 mg: 2-4 wks	14mg: 6wks, then 7mg: 2-4 wks.
Nicoderm	24 hrs. #14 box	21 mg: 6 wks, then 14 mg: 2 wks, then 7 mg: 2 wks	14 mg: 6 wks, then 7 mg: 2-4 wks
Prostep	24 hrs. #7/pkgs.	22 mg: 4-8 wks, then 11 mg: 2-4 wks	11 mg: 4-8 wks
Nicotrol	16 hrs. #14/box	15 mg: 4-12 wks, then 10 mg: 2-4 wks, then 5 mg: 2-4 wks	10 mg for patients with signs of nicotine excess

The **24** hour skin patches reduce early morning craving.
The **16** hour skin patch wears off at bedtime and so reduces nicotine induced sleep disturbances.

It has been proven that patients using these withdrawal systems are often successful if they can abstain from smoking the first two weeks. Failure is more frequent if smoking occurs during that time.

Caffeine (coffee)

Effects include: Alertness, energy, insomnia, diarrhea, and sometimes, rapid or premature heart beats.
                 Physical dependence can occur.
Withdrawl: Headache, fatigue, anxiety.

One cup of coffee has 85 mg caffeine; tea has 50 mg; cola (12 oz.) has 50 mg; and even chocolate has a small amount of caffeine. Half life is about 5 hours.

Anabolic Steroids (testosterone and its derivatives)

Mental effects: Initially euphoria, hyperactivity, irritability, hostility, violence ("roid rage"), anxiety, depression, and bodily complaints.

Withdrawl: Depression, anxiety, fatigue, suicidality, and insomnia.

These, in conjunction with exercise, cause increased muscle mass and physical performance. They have been abused extensively in most sports. Amounts taken are typically 10-40 times the medical dosages. Liver cancer is reported to occur in 1-7 years. 50% of users have reported hallucinations, paranoid delusions, mania, or depression (Reference 6). An increase in unhealthy cholesterol causes a 3-6-fold rise in coronary heart disease (hypertension, heart attacks, strokes). Male pattern baldness, body hair growth, acne, decreased testicular size, lower sperm count, breast enlargement, and prostate cancer can occur. Premature bone closure may cause adolescent users to be stunted and never reach their full adult height. Also headaches, dizziness, nosebleeds, stomach complaints, muscle cramps, tendon ruptures, and liver damage (yellow skin and eyes) can happen. A dependency pattern similar to heroin addiction has been reported. Sharing needles can spread AIDS. Dr Robert Kerr, author of The Practical Use of Anabolic Steroids with Athletes, stopped prescribing these because athletes would take more than he recommended (Reference 32). Physical health is seldom appreciated until it is lost.

> Labs: intensive training can alter liver enzymes (AST,ALT), but LDH5, and alkaline phosphatase can be measured to determine anabolic steroid effects. Glucose tolerance, thyroid hormones (and globulin) and testosterone decrease. Blood lipids worsen; HDL (high density lipoprotein) decreases, and the LDL/HDL ratio may increase 3 fold (persists up to 7 months after steroid stopped).

Hallucinogens (LSD, (lysergic acid diethylamide), psilocybin, mescaline)

Intoxication: Hallucinations, depersonalization, dilated pupils, high blood pressure and heart rate, uncoordination.

The effects of LSD are typically stopped within 1 hour by thorazine (chlorpromazine) 50mg IM. Valium 10mg by mouth or IM every 2 hours (maximum is 4 doses) can be helpful. For PCP or STP, thorazine is dangerous. Haldol 1-4 mg IM by mouth every 2 hours (with cogentin 1-2mg twice daily) until the patient is calm is safer for all hallucinogens.

Protocols 1-5 may be started when the patient is stable.

Volatile Hydrocarbons / Petroleum Derivatives

Glue, gasoline, varnish, paint thinner, lighter fluid, aerosols, benzene.

Intoxication: Slurred speech, hallucinations, psychosis, staggering, aromatic odor on breath, rapid heart rate and irregularity.

These can cause permanent brain damage and cardiac ventricular fibrillation. Liver, kidney and heart damage can occur. Liver enzymes can be checked, and Haldol 1-5mg every 6 hours (with cogentin 1-2mg twice daily) can be given until the patient is calm. Epinephrine should be avoided because of cardiac sensitization. Protocol 1-5 may be started when the patient is physically stable.

Belladonna Alkaloids

Over the counter atropine, homatropine hyoscyamine, scopolamine, stramonium, morning glory seeds.

For urinary retention, delirium, stupor, coma, fever and hypertension (then shock), give physostigmine (antilirium) 2mg IV every 20 minutes (rate no more than 1mg per minute). Watch for copious salivary secretion (reversal of dry mouth anticholinergic toxicity) and clearing of symptoms. Inderal (propranolol) can be used for rapid heart rate. Protocols 1-5 may be started when the patient is stable.

Intoxication: Confusion, dry mouth, blurred vision, dilated pupils, difficulty swallowing.

Urine Drug Testing	
Substance	Tests Positive in Urine for:
Alcohol	7-12 hours
Benzodiazapine	3 days
Barbiturate	24 hours (short half life) 3 weeks (long half life)
Quaalude	7 days
Amphetamine	48 hours
Cocaine	6-8 hours, metabolites 2-4 days
Heroin	36-72 hours
Methadone	3 days
Morphine	48-72 hours
Propoxyphene (Darvon)	6-48 hours
Codeine	48 hours
Cannabis (Marijuana)	3-28 days (according to use)
PCP	8 days

Substances of abuse can be detected in the urine.

[Reference 4]

121

THE PSYCHIATRIC STANDARD AND THIS METHOD - BALANCING THE TWO

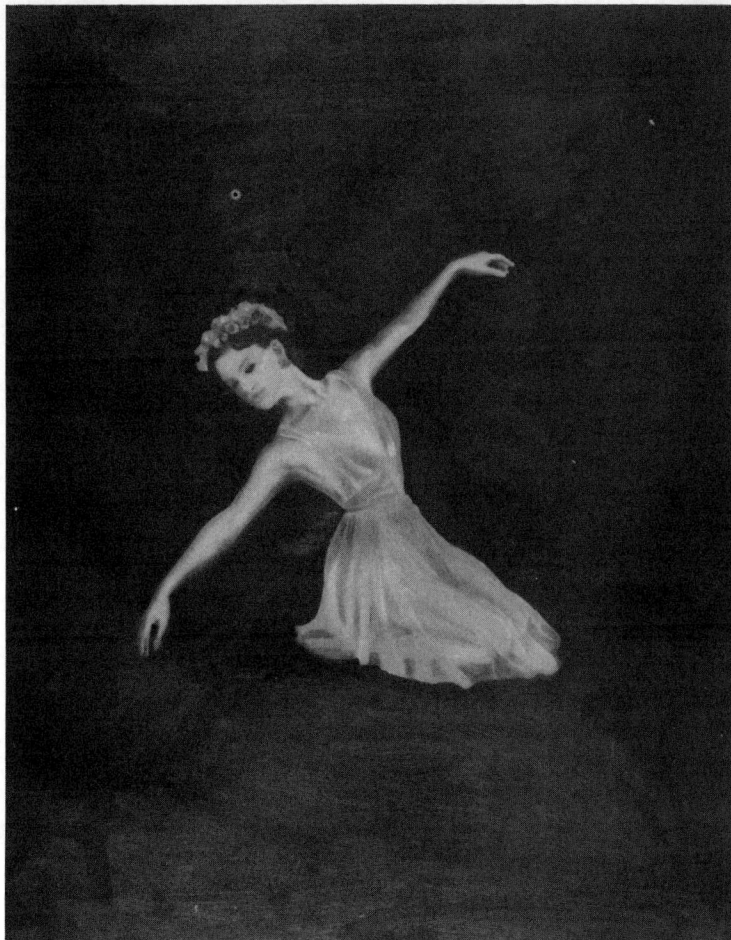

*Except for cases of obvious psychosis, I prefer to use the protocol method before the standard method. **Out of respect for the current system and the concept that new ideas complement proven tradition, the standard approaches are outlined below.***

This a review of what standard psychiatry offers. It is specified when my method is significantly different from standard treatments. The protocol method can be used before or when standard options have failed.

*It is best to **try one medication at a time**, in order to tell what is helping.*

Panic (Anxiety) Treatment

■ **ANTIDEPRESSANTS**: Should also be called "Anti-Panics", because they are a primary treatment. According to research if adequate dosage is maintained long enough almost all patients "clear". The first several weeks of treatment patients may feel they are worse with increased panic. Xanax, or a beta blocker such as Inderol can relieve this. Antidepressant dosage is increased as tolerated, about every other day, until a full dose is reached. Standard psychiatry says adrenaline like side effects are temporary and cause patients to flee treatment that could have fixed them within 3-6 weeks. Indeed, some panic disorder patients have an excess of norepinephrine receptors (see glossary) in the brain that is reduced to normal in three to four weeks, by this method of treatment. My hypothesis is that antidepressant adverse reactions:

-sometimes are simply **side-effects**

-or can represent **excess NE receptors**

-but often mean **contributing factors (manic depression, psychosis, ADHD, GABA, or thyroid malfunction*)** are present and cause the panic disorder. The antidepressants for panic usually react adversely with and worsen these conditions.

*(NE or electrical instability, dopamine elevation, DA/NE failure, GABA or thyroid malfunction.)

PROVEN ANTIDEPRESSANTS: STANDARD TREATMENT

> Tofranil 10-25mg at bedtime.
> or Norpramine 10-25mg in morning.
> or Pamelar 10mg at bedtime.

Tofranil and Pamelar are favorites when insomnia is present. Dosages can be raised as tolerated to an average of 150mg for the first two and 75mg for Pamelar, for 3-6 weeks treatment.

PROMISING ANTIDEPRESSANTS: STANDARD TREATMENT

> Zoloft 50 mg: 1/2-1 in A.M.
> Paxil 20 mg: 1/2-1 in A.M.
> Prozac 10-20 mg in A.M.

These serotonin enhancers are especially good in perfectionistic, critical and orderly people. If a serotonin correction helps panic I call this a **low serotonin panic disorder**. Some of the original antidepressants (Elavil, Sinequan) can help, but tend to be sedating and can cause weight gain. Yet some people need this. Other antidepressants are questionably helpful. If serotonin antidepressants fail, a norepinephrine one (Norpramine) can be tried. Wellbutrin (75mg twice daily), also corrects NE and may help some panic victims that have mild features of ADHD (DA/NE failure). If a NE antidepressant fixes the panic I call this a **low NE panic disorder.**

MAOI ANTIDEPRESSANTS: STANDARD TREATMENT

Nardil starting at 15 mg daily can be increased by 15 mg weekly to a maximum of 90 mg per day. These are according to many sources more effective than the other antidepressants. Many doctors prescribe this medication freely, but I avoid it as a first choice because of **dangerous** side-effects (stroke) if the wrong food is eaten. A **strict diet** must be followed. Also, other antidepressants need to be out of the system before MAOI is started: Specifically Prozac for 5 weeks, Zoloft and Paxil for 3 weeks, and all others for 2 weeks. It can also be dangerous to combine an MAOI with Ritalin or other stimulants, which should be out of the system before MAOI is started.

Occasionally any antidepressant can cause a **strong adverse emotional reaction**, usually within hours to days which I term **"Reactivity"**. This can be relieved with a 4% dopamine reduction using:

Stelazine 2 mg

The broken/bitten or cut tablet can be kept on the tongue for 30-60 seconds before swallowing with water. Discomfort usually clears within 1-2 minutes. If further comfort is needed, Xanax 0.25-0.5 mg is effective.

If intolerance towards an antidepressant continues, the dosage cannot be raised due to severe side-effects. As distress levels worsen hour by hour, or day by day, to a degree dopamine reduction antidotes are required, suspicion should grow that a **different antidepressant or protocol 2-5 medication is needed.** Whether NE receptors are excessive becomes less relevant than the reactivity in the brain, which precludes treatment by that S or NE antidepressant. In treating panic, a goal is to force the NE receptor volume down by providing antidepressant, yet sometimes we cannot because adverse antidepressant reactions are too strongly present. A decision is then made either to continue the antidepressant at a lower dose, so NE receptors can be gradually reduced and anxiety fixed, or to discontinue the antidepressant. Note that as the antidepressant dose is being raised, the underlying reactivity may interfere with results. An ideal non-destabilizing NE correction may sometimes be attained by keeping the antidepressant dose low.

I routinely give one antidote pill (Stelazine) with or without Xanax at the start of each different antidepressant trial to protect patients from possible adverse reaction.

■ BENZODIAZEPINES: STANDARD TREATMENT

These are medications which can be added to antidepressant treatment, especially during the initial phases when the antidepressant can worsen anxiety. These medications are rapidly effective, providing relief from panic within minutes to an hour. At lower doses addiction risk is minimal. A goal would be to discontinue the "benzo" as soon as the antidepressant (or any other medication) is effectively clearing the panic. This medication should be tapered gently. Occasionally however, this is the only medication to help anxiety, and in that situation it should be continued. These people have a defect in their GABA system, that GABA correctors neutralize. 75-90% of the brain's neurons have GABA. The following, in order of preference, are benzodiazepines most commonly successful for panic, with low dosage guidelines.

> **XANAX 0.25-0.5 mg tablets:** 1/2-1 tablet three times per day as needed. Mainstream psychiatry makes allowances for up to 6-10mg per day. My "comfort cut-off" is 1.5 mg per day because I worry that other chemistry needs correcting, not anesthetizing, and that higher doses of any benzodiazepine place people at increased risk of auto accidents. Yet situations exist where higher range Xanax is needed.

> **KLONOPIN 0.5-1 mg tablets:** 1/2-1 tablet usually at bedtime because it helps sleep and lasts 24 hours.

OTHER MISCELLANEOUS AGENTS: STANDARD TREATMENT

INDERAL: 80 mg per day in divided doses, up to 160 mg per day within 1 week is especially useful and **comforting for rapid heart rate, palpitations**, tremor, sweating, and may partially help panic. Since this medicine is not for asthmatics, diabetics, or people with congestive heart failure, less effective other beta blockers are used cautiously (Metoprolol, Atenolol - "tenormin", etc.) in those situations.

TENORMIN 25 mg: 1/2-1 tablet once or twice daily. This is another beta blocker with a longer half life (7 hours) then inderal (4 hours), It has been more helpful than inderal for some patients. It too is a blood pressure medicine.

BUSBAR: 5-20 mg TID for at least 2 weeks sometimes works for anxiety, but rarely for more severe panic. It is essentially nontoxic and may have antidepressant qualities (mild serotonin enhancement).

ANTIHISTAMINES: Results occur by sedation. Includes Benadryl (10-25mg) or Atarax (10-50mg) 4 times a day.

NEUROLEPTICS: Low dose Thorazine or Mellaril (10-25mg) 3-4 times per day can help and also sedate.

COGNITIVE THERAPY: May help for avoidance after medical stabilization of panic is doNE

MY METHOD: Use Protocol 2-5 if antidepressants and benzodiazepines have been unsuccessful. The GABA agent (benzodiazepine) may be continued during the protocols if necessary for comfort. Useful clues can be obtained with short sequential medication trials. Blending can be done later after the medications are rated individually. Patients may have a fraction of disturbance in several systems.

The electrical smoothers, **Depakote** (or less often **Tegretal**) may work and are gaining acceptance as helpful in atypical panic attacks. Sometimes they work only temporarily. The cause in that circumstance is usually DA/NE failure, or GABA malfunction.

The NE stabilizer **Lithium,** according to the literature, doesn't help panic, but in practice often works completely (see page 53). Suicidal thinking, emotionality, creativity, and family backgrounds of high achievement can be present for these people.

Dopamine reducers such as **Stelazine** in low dose normalize a few panic disorders.

DA/NE replacement by **Ritalin** or another stimulant sometimes clears the most resistant panic disorders, yet low dose simultaneous dopamine reduction is necessary 21% of the time. These patients may have had difficulty concentrating, disliked math, and disliked practically all other psychotropic medicines.

GABA malfunction is occasionally the main problem. These patients may have adverse reactions to most psychotropic medications similar to DA/NE failure (ADD) patients, but stimulant worsens these patients. I pick the benzodiazepine that works best in the lowest dose possible. Like Ritalin for ADD, it appears GABA agents can be taken long term in low dose without tolerance or addiction if a person truly has major GABA malfunction. Alternatively an MAOI can be attempted. Standard psychiatry may be over-utilizing GABA agents (such as Xanax, Ativan, and Valium) while missing some minor chemical imbalance that, when corrected, could have made the brain medically normal, rather than anesthetized.

Mild **thyroid** dysfunction is a common cause of panic and of adverse medication reactions. Thyroid medicine helps some, but typically anxiety is fixed best with other medications. Thyroid medication corrects primarily fatigue and weight gain. **Estrogen occasionally has fixed a resistant panic disordered female.**

There are at least 2 broad types of depression: serotonin and norepinephriNE Antidepressants are the primary treatment to correct deficiencies in these brain transmitter chemicals (S and NE), or their receptors. Normal levels of these substances in the brain allow the person to feel normal. The medicines block reabsorption of the transmitter substance into nerves, so more is left working and felt. The medicines are not narcotic or addictive, and are being designed safer. Many patients report relief occurring the same day treatment starts, yet others may have results delayed up to 6 weeks. The degree of response occurring within 2 weeks often correlates with outcome. If the medication is activating, prescribe it for the morning, if it is sedating, give it at bedtime. If sedation (or activation) is problematic, causing daytime grogginess (or nighttime insomnia), lower the dose or change the medication.

What follows is standard depression treatment, followed by my approach.

Standard Depression Treatment:

   1. **SSRI** (serotonin enhancer) - A 4-6 week trial of Zoloft, Paxil, or Prozac.

   2. If above fails, change to any other antidepressant, especially towards the norepinephrine enhancers (Tofranil, Pamelar, Norpramine, Wellbutrin, etc.).

   3. If above fails, add a mood stabilizer (Lithium, Depakote, or Tegretal).

   4. If above fails, change to MAOI (more powerful yet more dangerous); before starting MAOI, Prozac must be stopped at least 5 weeks prior, and Zoloft or Paxil stopped 2-3 weeks prior.

   5. If above fails, add Lithium, or low dose thyroid.

   6. If above fails, discontinue MAOI for 2 weeks, start a TCA (tricyclic standard antidepressant), and add MAOI or SSRI slowly.

   7. If above fails, antidepressant is combined with antipsychotic medication.

   8. ETC (electric shock therapy).

MY METHOD: In my practice, #1 and #2 are the steps I take. I compress the SSRI's into Protocol #1.

Concerning steps #3-7, I feel uncomfortable blending medications before knowing what each can do alone Concerning step #3, manic depressive chemistry usually destabilizes with antidepressants, so why add manic depressive medications (lithium, Depakote, or Tegretal) to an antidepressant? The problem is delicate. For example: Sometimes Tegretal alone causes destabilization with manic depressive chemistry because the structure of Tegretal resembles a tricyclic antidepressant. Occasionally, a very low dose of a serotonin antidepressant can be added to a mood stabilizer to help depression.

Concerning step #5, even thyroid medicine can be destabilizing for the protocol 2 disorders and so should be tried, if possible, alone Unfortunately, thyroid works slowly and commits treatment to weeks of not trying multiple other options, so I leave this for last, after most of the brain chemistry has been solved. Thyroid helps fatigue, weight, and only occasionally depression. Cytomel tends to work in 1-2 days.

Concerning step #7, what if the antidepressant is aggravating an underlying elevated dopamine (psychosis) chemistry? Again it is wisest to first try the dopamine reducer ("antipsychotic") medicine alone.

Instead of following steps #3-8, I prefer to make sure both NE and S antidepressants have been tried, as well as protocols 2-5. This solves practically all depression cases, i.e. they did not look manic depressive, psychotic, or hyperactive (ADHD) but were chemically responsive in those categories.

Concerning steps #4 and #6, I am avoidant of MAOI's because of the dietary restrictions and stroke risk, yet am willing to prescribe them as a last resort, at which time they usually work well.

Traditionally, if **children** were treated, they received TCA's such as Tofranil, Norpramine, or Elavil. This had some degree of cardiac risk. Children should not be given more than 3mg/kg/day of a TCA. It will be interesting to see if the safer SSRI'S will be used to treat children. I have occasionally, and successfully, used Zoloft, Paxil, Effexor, Luvox, Prozac, or Serzone in chemically imbalanced children at the same dosage their parent required.

MANIC DEPRESSION (BIPOLAR DISORDER) TREATMENT

My method and standard treatment are similar.

Mood stabilizer medications include lithium which smooths NE instability, and "anti-convulsants" which smooth electricity (Depakote, Tegretol).

- **Lithium** responsive patients most frequently are characterized by mood problems, profound **emotional pain** levels (suicidal thoughts, crying), **creativity** (musicians, artists, poets) and **impulsivity**. Sometimes these people have cluster headaches. Mild, easily correctable NE instability can occur in some very successful people.

- **Depakote** responsive patients most frequently are characterized by **anxiety**, uncomfortable **moods**, and **sometimes headaches**.

- **Tegretal** helps physically explosive patients who feel more **frustration** or **rage** and less depression. Some heroin or cocaine **addicts** are transitioned nicely from their habit using Tegretol, especially if they normally were hyperactive or agitated.

> *Medically these three groups of patients usually destabilize (deteriorate) on antidepressants. The adrenergic NE antidepressants typically induce decompensation more than the serotonin anti-depressants.*

Treatment depends on symptom severity as well as the above mentioned subtype characteristics. The following options are available:

1. **Lithium** alone: 300 mg, 2-3 times daily
2. **Lithium and neuroleptic**, if the patient is somewhat psychotic (for example: Mellaril 25-50 mg every two hours as needed) or
   Lithium and benzodiazepine if the patient is somewhat anxious (for example: ativan 1-2 mg every 4-6 hours).
3. **Tegretol** (100 mg 2-3 times per day) and/or
   Depakote (125-250 mg three times per day) alone, or with above.
4. **ECT** - an option according to mainstream psychiatry.

MY METHOD: Again, I prefer to **give one medication at a time** so efficacy can be clarified. Blends can then follow. If someone is too psychotic, neuroleptic (a dopamine reducer) alone is usually helpful:

Haldol 5mg: 3 times per day
Cogentin 1mg: 3 times per day to prevent side effects

If that doesn't work, a different class of neuroleptic often does (see page 70)

According to standard psychiatry, **ETC** has been shown to be helpful in manic patients who are somewhat psychotic. However, I prefer to give those patients a dopamine reducer medicine, or medication, if it works, from any of the protocols.

Concerning medications for manic depression, I believe over-utilization of lab tests interferes with quick trial and error sampling that so frequently is successful. If a medication is successful, I usually order the routine labs.

See the Medication Toxicity chapter for more information on lithium blood levels.

It is sometimes recommended to combine antidepressants and standard mood stabilizers (lithium, Tegretol, Depakote). My experience is the **NE antidepressants** are highly **destabilizing** of manic depressive chemistry. The serotonin antidepressants are sometimes helpful, but may feed into NE or electrical systems that are unstable (affiliated too close to dopamine), which then results in further destabilization. The Stelazine antidote is helpful in these situations.

Klonopin (clonazepam) structurally resembles a benzodiazepine. It may have a slight anti-manic depressive action because of its electricity smoothing "anticonvulsant" effects. Because sedation can occur, this is usually taken at bedtime. Occasional manic depressives who could not take other medications did well with Klonopin 2 mg three times per day. For seizure disorders, 20 mg per day can be used. I try to limit dosage to 2 mg or less per day because of possible addiction risk at higher dose ranges. Klonopin 1-2 mg is about equal to a glass of wine. Some patients take only half of the smallest Klonopin (0.5 mg tablet) to avoid sedation.
If an antidepressant worked nicely, but then destabilized, adding any mood stabilizer, including gentle Klonopin may correct the situation.

SCHIZOPHRENIA (Psychosis) TREATMENT

It is important to remove any underlying organic factors that could cause psychosis. Genetics, structural, and functional abnormalities in the brain cause schizophrenia. Heredity, viral infection during fetal development, and prematurity are the most common causes of schizophrenia.

Medication is highly effective in relieving symptoms, usually within hours. The longer dopamine elevation (psychosis) is left untreated, the longer and higher the medication dose will need to be before results occur. The choice of neuroleptic can be tailored to personal needs (see chart). Haldol is good for severe psychosis if alertness is preferred. (2-5mg every 4 hours as needed). Thorazine is sedating and good if violence is occurring. Mellaril can help resistant insomnia (10mg:1-3 or 25mg:1-2 at bedtime).

If an **antipsychotic is failing, switch to a different class** (see A-J on chart on page 70). If all classes have failed, try Clozaril (clozapine). Though tardive dyskinesia is not a risk, agranulocytosis is and makes weekly blood monitoring mandatory. If a patient is **noncompliant**, long acting shots can be given:

Haldol decanoate, 50-100mg IM (range 50-300) every 2-5 weeks.
or
Prolixin decanoate, 25mg IM (range 6.25-100mg) every 3-6 weeks

---

When the patient is stable, consider reducing the dose.
> **Lithium** helps as many as 50% of schizophrenic looking patients.
> **Benzodiazepines** (klonapin) may be helpful if anxiety is prominent.
> **Tegretal** can be helpful, especially if the patient is violent.

Electroconvulsive therapy has not been proven effective in chronic schizophrenia.

Causes:

There are many hidden conditions that can cause DA/NE failure (ADHD). A variety of subtle brain injuries developmentally or later in life (stroke, aging) can cause this. The list includes fetal, infantile, and toddler brain stresses such as head trauma, fever, viral inflammations, and prematurity. Heredity also can be a cause of ADHD. Aids victims can be emotionally comforted by DA/NE replacement. Some severe herpes suffers (temporal lobe injured) also respond positively with this treatment when all other methods had failed. Some people are resistant to their own thyroid hormone, and have ADHD 46% of the time. Severe DA/NE failure victims usually have an injury factor combining with a genetic one to cause disability.

Theory:

The chemical defect is an underactivity of dopamine/norepinephrine causing low blood flow to several areas of the brain. Stimulant treatment corrects failed DA/NE resulting in a reversal of the low blood flow problem. The stimulant however can elevate DA in another area of the brain causing psychotic agitation. Thus DA reducing (blocking) antipsychotic is often required during treatment with a stimulant.

Clinical:

DA/NE failure is a very commonly missed diagnosis in adults because symptoms are usually ill defined. Vague symptoms include anxiety, distress, depression, and confusion or psychosis. **This disorder is characterized by the most bad medication reactions of any psychiatric diagnosis except for some GABA malfunction patients** (See graph on pagea 64). This may include worsening and destabilization from serotonin antidepressants (for example: Prozac, and Elavil), sometimes NE antidepressants (for example: Norpramine), Buspar and usually Lithium. One antidepressant, **Wellbutrin**, structurally resembles a weak stimulant, and is sometimes the proper match for a mild ADHD situation in an adult. Because it is not an amphetamine, it can be tried before advancing to full DA/NE replacement treatment. Concerning medication reactions, moderate or eventual worsening may occur with electrical stabilizers (Depakote, Tegretol) and dopamine reducers (for example: Mellaril, Stelazine). Even GABA agents (for example: Xanax, Valium, Ativan) by negative feedback on NE sometimes aggravates DA/NE failure.

Different stimulants should be tested one at a time to attain the best match for replacement treatment. The wrong stimulant can also cause adverse reactions. If a stimulant initially works, then destabilizes, it may work by being blended with a low dose dopamine reducer.

ADULTS:

CHOICES FOR DA/NE REPLACEMENT	DOSE RANGE
Wellbutrin	75mg at 8 A.M., 2 P.M., up to 150 mg - 8 A.M., 2, 8 P.M.
Cylert	37.5mg in A.M., up to 112.5 mg in A.M.
Tenuate	25 mg 2-3 times a day
Ionamin	15 mg-60 mg in A.M.
Ritalin	5 mg-20 mg at 8 A.M., 12, 4 P.M.
Dexedrine	5 mg-20 mg at 8 A.M., 12, 4 P.M.

See protocol 3 on page 43 for treatment information, and graph on page 73

FAVORITE CHOICES FOR DOPAMINE REDUCTION	DOSE RANGE:	FEATURE:
Mellaril...........	10mg 2-3 at Bedtime	Sleeper
OR	25mg 1-2 at Bedtime	
Stelazine..........	1-2mg in AM daily	Alertness

CHILDREN:

FDA approval is for Ritalin, Dexedrine, and Cylert. See the explanation on page 44.

If **Ritalin** is ineffective at the child's full dose, switching to the same dose of **Dexedrine** may work since this is stronger.

Clondine with stimulant or alone may help frustration and explosiveness (see page 73).

If it doesn't work, the more effective stimulant can be blended with the dopamine reducer Mellaril.

For children aged 2-12, **Mellaril** can be given up to **3mg/kg/day.** A starting dose is 10mg, 2-3 times per day with stimulant doses.

"ADHD" children by puberty sometimes **differentiate** into manic depression. Either condition can cause hyperactivity. Yet the NE unstable children (manic depressive) have more adverse reactions to stimulants.

OTHER MEDICATIONS: NONE?

For severe ADHD, antidepressants (Norpamine, Tofranil, Wellbutrin) are not as good. They, in fact, frequently worsen symptoms. In children, Norpramine or Tofranil are more dangerous to the heart, and Wellbutrin has seizure risk. **Stimulants are safer and more effective**. The MAOI Tranylcypromine is more dangerous and has major dietary restrictions.

DA/NE replacement treatment is an attempt to match medium or mild strength stimulants to structurally similar brain norepinephriNE **"Street" methamphetamine** is abused by addicts and resembles epineph-rine which is 25 times more powerful than NE. NE is in the brain and regulates normal functioning. Epinephrine is in the adrenal gland and is used during emergencies. Addiction and tolerance do not occur in replacement treatment, but are a problem when "normal" people take amphetamines; these patients will feel "hyper", "speedy", and insomniac. DA/NE failure patients given amphetamine (that is matched to their chemistry) feel normal, but possibly insomniac. Therefore, doses are given not too late in the day.

The risk of toxic psychosis exists not only for the stimulants, but antidepressants, lithium, anticonvulsants, neuroleptics, thyroid medicine, and even benzodiazepines.

Misuse of methylphenidate does not appear to be a problem in patients under adequate medical supervi-sion when recommended dose levels are maintained, but the drug should be given cautiously to patients, with a history of substance abuse.

When DA/NE failure coexists with another chemical imbalance, the best medicine from any other proto-col can usually be combined with the ADD/ADHD treatment.

Manic depressive (NE or electrically unstable) and psychotic (dopamine toxic) people tend to get much worse on stimulant. If one of these conditions is mixed with DA/NE failure (i.e. ADHD plus manic depression, ADHD plus psychosis), the best matched stimulant can be blended with a dopamine reducer or perhaps Lithium.

When ADHD and bipolar co-exist, stimulant might help for months, but then can destabilize the NE instability to cause a toxic psychosis. Stopping the stimulant 2 days while giving anti-adrenergic medi-cines (page 49) allows a "washout" so treatment can resume. Thus, stimulants are tricky and potentially treacherous. The practically miraculous result they can offer to "DA/NE failure" conditions makes trying this worthwhile. Unfortunately, the amphetamines have been discovered and re-discovered in different times and places as a key to productivity and happiness, only to lead to social anguish and disappoint-ment. The medical uses as described above are wonderful exceptions to the dark side of stimulants.

MEDICATION TOXICITY LABS - REFERENCE

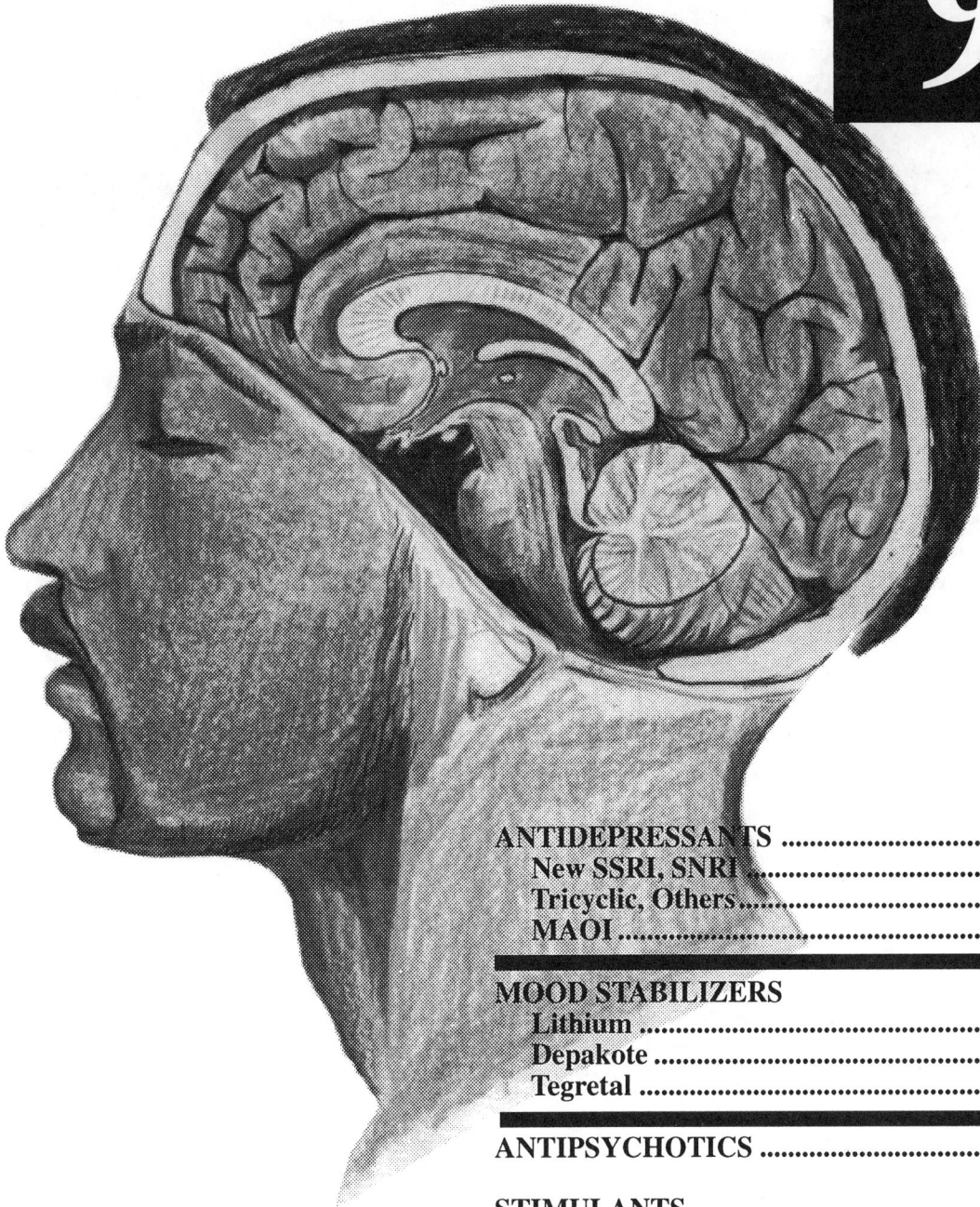

This chapter, like a car's seat belt, is for your protection; and just like car accidents, things can go wrong. By knowing about your medicine, you are likely to do well concerning risks. Actual dangerous occurrences with these medications are rare. Comparable to a car, these brain transmitter correctors have much to offer for civilization. The medication information insert you get with your prescription provides an exhaustive but complete compilation of toxic possibilities. The information which follows is approximate.

ANTIDEPRESSANT

Three broad categories of antidepressants are:
1. Selective serotonin reuptake inhibitors (SSRI's) and
   Selective serotonin, norepinephrine reuptake inhibitors (SNRI's)
2. Tricyclic and heterocyclic antidepressants (TCA, HCA)
3. Monoamine oxidase inhibitors (MAOI's)

Diagnostic Destabilization Symptoms from Antidepressants:

Important adverse reactions can occur from any class of antidepressant, and may signify a different underlying chemistry is present. This can be any factor from the ten medical access points to the brain, i.e, manic depression, psychosis, ADHD, anxiety or thyroid disturbed chemistries. This can result in emotional or physical worsening, or in accentuation of normal side effects.

Sometimes switching to a different antidepressant will help. Yet, **as each new antidepressant again causes adverse reactions in the patient, suspicions grow** that antidepressants are destabilizing (worsening) some underlying chemistry and **that another protocol is needed** to identify and correct this.

ANTIDEPRESSANT DESTABILIZATION

Emotional Destabilization triggered by antidepressants include any of the following: Patients may feel worse, more anxious, confused, labile, distressed, dazed, "in a fog", fatigued, exhausted, weak, shaky, "hyper", agitated, violent, suicidal, scattered with thinking, dulled, "zombied", like crying, bizarrely elated, wired", or "amped". Also the medication may have worked then stopped working despite increasing dosage. They can have nightmares or hallucinations. Presenting complaints may intensify. One antidepressant may cause problems while another does not.

Somatic (Physical) Destabilization triggered by antidepressants may include any of the following: rapid heart rate, palpitations, diarrhea, headaches, sweating, restless legs, flushing, speech impairment, or increased craving for whatever addiction was their problem (food, alcohol, drugs, etc.). Weight gain with a weight loss type of antidepressant can also be an example of this. Extreme levels of physical side-effects (nausea, headaches, etc.) raises suspicion that physical destabilization is occurring. Sedation by an activating antidepressant is also usually destabilization.

This vaguely defined antidepressant adverse reaction I call **"Reactivity"**, until it is exactly defined by the protocols. These reactions can be used as diagnostic clues to guide treatment.

Yet some of these reactions can just be side effects. See what follows for medical effects of the antidepressants, and the graph on page 68 to see the differences between the three broad categories of antidepressants.

1. NEW ANTIDEPRESSANTS: SSRI's, SNRI's

SSRI - Selective serotonin reuptake inhibitor
SNRI - Selective Serotonin, norepinephrine reuptake inhibitor

Medicines have been designed that are practically harmless. They are very selective in correcting a particular brain transmitter abnormality. If an SSRI or SNRI is helpful but has side effects, switching to a different one often corrects the problem.

Some people, for example the elderly, have to be on many medications due to physical illness. Effexor does not occupy enzyme systems (cytochrome P-450-2D6) as much and so is a safer choice for these people.

SIDE EFFECT	ZOLOFT	PAXIL	LUVOX	PROZAC	EFFEXOR
Nausea	26%	26%	40%	21%	37%
Anorexia	3	6	6	9	11
Dry Mouth	16	18	14	10	22
Constipation	8	14	10	5	15
Diarrhea	18	12	11	12	8
Nervousness	3	5	12	15	13
Tremor	11	8	5	8	5
Sweating	8	11	7	8	12
Dizziness	12	13	11	6	19
Insomnia	16	13	21	14	18
Fatigue	10	15	?	4	12
Somnolence	13	23	22	12	23
Vision Disturbance	4	4	3	3	9
Male Sexual Dysfunction	16	13	8	2	12
Female Sexual Dysfunction	2	2	2	2	2

Possible Medical Effects from Antidepressants

2. TRICYLIC and clinically similar compounds can have activation or sedation, dryness of mouth, dizziness, cardiac effects, seizure risk and weight gain. (See the medication graph on page 68). Doses can be divided into several doses per day to minimize side effects. If sedation is occurring, the medicine should be taken all at bedtime.

Anticholinergic (dry mouth):

Dry mouth, constipation, and blurring can occur.
Most of these decrease in 1-2 weeks.

The elderly can get confused due to anticholinergic effects. The medication graph can be used to pick a less anticholinergic antidepressant.

Other side effects are rare and include painful narrow angle glaucoma in the eye, urinary hesitancy/ retention, rapid heart rate, mental clouding, speech blockage, and impaired memory.

Cardiovascular

Dizziness and lowering of blood pressure can cause falls and injury, especially in the elderly. Standing up slowly, increasing medication doses slowly or switching to a safer antidepressant (see graph) can correct this.

Rapid heart rate is an anticholinergic effect. Picking from the graph a medicine with less of this can correct the problem. Some people are especially vulnerable and require Inderal or Tenormen to stop this. Often the heart rate acceleration is a sign of destabilization, and may indicate the wrong medication is being used.

The TCA's help decrease premature beats. Conduction ECG changes include prolongation of the PR interval, QT, or QRS widening, ST depression and T-wave changes.

TCA's should be avoided if bundle branch block is present. With second and third degree blocks, fatality can occur.

A QT interval exceeding 0.440 seconds (corrected for rate) is associated with increased serious cardiac risk. (Reference 10, page 103).

Suppression of heart function with congestive heart failure and ankle swelling, can occur especially in the elderly. Overdoses can kill by making the heart irregular.

Seizures are more likely to occur from excess Wellbutrin, Anafranil, or Ludiomil, but also with any TCA/ HCA overdose. Epileptics who normally may have seizures are more at risk. People abruptly withdrawing from alcohol or sedative hypnotics (valium type medicines) also are more likely to have a seizure.

Painful and persistent **erection** can occur from desyrel once in 0.5% of male patients. This is not dose related and is an emergency. Treatment is to stop the medicine, and contact a urologist immediately.

3. MAOI's are the most dangerous antidepressants. Eating the wrong food, or combining this medicine with another medicine can cause **elevation in blood pressure and possible stroke.**

At risk medications include:
Various decongestants and cold formulas containing Ephedrine, Phenylephrine, Phenylpropanolamine, Pseudoephedrine.
Asthma medications (epinephrine, ephedrine).
Antihypertensive medicines.
Narcotics - Meperidine (Demerol).
Amphetamines, cocaine, crack.
Dopa
Buspar (Buspirone).

At risk foods contain tyramine:
Aged cheeses (cheddar, English stilton, blue, swiss, etc.) cause 80% of all "hypertensive crises".
Cottage cheese, processed sliced cheese, ricotta, cream cheeses and yogurt are safe.
Chianti wine, fava beans, concentrated yeast extracts(brewer's is safe), pickled herring, aged meat-sausages, sauerkraut, aspartamine artificial sweetener greater than 1 gram/day, and soy sauce.

Other effects MAOI's can cause are:
Low blood pressure, dizziness.
Liver toxicity once every 3-10 thousand patients.
Weight gain, narrow angle glaucoma, urinary retention, diminished orgasms. They are less anticho-linergic than TCA's.

The MAOI diet and medication restrictions should continue for 2 weeks after a MAOI is stopped. A different antidepressant, stimulant, or thyroid medicine should not be started until 2 weeks after the MAOI is stopped.

Also, other antidepressants need to be out of the system before MAOI is started: Specifically Prozac for 5 weeks, Zoloft and Paxil for 3 weeks, and all others for 2 weeks. It can also be dangerous to combine an MAOI with Ritalin or other stimulants, which should be out of the system before MAOI is started.

Lab Work for Antidepressants

A plasma level can be obtained, 10-14 hours after the last dose for Prozac, Elavil, Norpramine, Pamelar, or Tofranil. This can help concerning further dosage decisions if the medicine is not working after at least one week of a steady dose.

MAO Platelet inhibition for MAOI's can be measured, but the clinical usefulness of this requires further study. Many labs do not offer this test. Liver function tests can be useful for MAOI's. (Reference 10, page 115).

LITHIUM DESTABILIZATION

Mental Worsening can occur from a low dose of lithium. This can be characterized by **distress, agitation, confusion, loss of coordination, sedation,** or an accentuation of normal side effects. This usually means lithium is the wrong medication.

POSSIBLE MEDICAL EFFECTS FROM LITHIUM:

Small doses usually have no problems.
Adverse reactions are usually dose related.

VARIOUS LITHIUM BLOOD LEVELS

LITHIUM 1.5 MEG/L OR LESS	1.5-2 MEG/L	2.0 MEG OR MORE
Side Effects	Early Toxicity	Toxicity
Drinking more fluid 38%	Nausea, vomiting	Heart arrhythmias
Fine hand tremor 37%	Diarrhea	Muscle jerks
Memory problems 32%	Severe tremor	Seizures
Increased urination 31%	Sluggish	Stupor, delirium
Weight gain 30%	Staggering, dizzy	Coma
Mental worsening 23%	Speech difficulties	Less urine,
ECG changes 20%		Kidney failure
Dizziness 20%		Death
Nausea 15%		
Diarrhea 14%	Rx: Stop, then	
Fluid retention 10%	Lower lithium	Rx: Stop lithium,
Hypothyroidism 8%-30%	Dose	Treat symptoms

Nausea 15%: Take lithium with food, **lower** or spread doses out, try slow release brand, or lithium citrate, or raise lithium doses more slowly. Drink some water to dilute the lithium in case of dehydration.

Diarrhea 14%: Lower the lithium dose, take lithium with meals, switch to lithium citrate, or take antidiarrheal medicine. Bentyl (20mg) 2 to 4 times/day. Slow release lithium may worsen diarrhea.

Weight Gain 30%: Lower the lithium dose, diet, and check for low thyroid clinically and with labs. Treat this if it is present. If it is fluid retention, spironolactone, 50mg 1-2x/day can carefully be used (may increase potassium). All options in the protocols may need explored for alterative agents.

Thyroid 8%-30%: Hypothyroid clinical signs or abnormal **thyroid** functions may occur. Increased TSH is the most sensitive test. Synthroid 50mcg, or Cytomel 25mcg may need added and adjusted, or lithium may be stopped if this is clinically possible. (Thyroid functions usually return to normal).

Parathyroid: Serum **calcium** and parathormone levels can increase in 10%, but this is rarely important. Symptoms theoretically include aggressiveness, confusion, psychosis, dementia and seizures.

Heart: ECG: "QRS wider, t-wave inverted or flat". Heart **irregularity** can cause palpitations or fainting. Rare sudden death is usually due to pre-existing heart disease. I have never seen this.

Kidneys: In 9 years, I have never seen either of these conditions. **Nephrogenic diabetes insipidus** - This is characterized by increased **urine volume** (4-8 liters/day), **increased serum lithium, sodium** and **low potassium** due to a difficulty concentrating urine. The treatment is to stop or lower the lithium to a once per day dose. Fluids are encouraged. Adding Amiloride 5-10mg twice daily (a diuretic) helps, and does not effect the lithium or electrolytes. **Interstitial cystitis** may happen from long term lithium treatment. A sudden rise in **serum creatinine** signifies this. It is usually reversible by stopping lithium.

White Blood Cell Count: This can **increase** from 12,500 to 15,000/mm3. is reversible and harmless.

Acne: This occasionally may appear or worsen with lithium. Tetracycline 250mg twice daily may control this as maintenance if necessary, or lithium may be stopped.

Psoriasis: This if pre-existing can be aggravated.

Hair loss: This rarely occurs, usually in women, and regrows by stopping the lithium. Low thyroid can cause hair loss.

Tremor 37%: This usually disappears after 2-3 weeks of lithium treatment. Lower more frequent doses may stop the tremor. Long acting lithium can produce less tremor. Other medicines can be added:
>   Propranolol(**Inderal**) **10-20mg 3-4 times per day.** Do not use this if congestive heart failure or
>   bronchospasm are present. Alternatives are
>   Metoprolol 25-50mg or Nadolol 20-40mg twice daily.

Seizures: These are rare, and usually in patients who have epilepsy.

Memory Problems 32%: Reducing the lithium dose may be necessary. Adding Mellaril 25mg at bedtime daily helps some (mild lithium organicity?). Switching to Tegretal may help (to improve vasopressin which lithium inhibits). Adding thyroid (synthroid 25mcg) may help or adding Folate 400ug daily may help.

LAB WORK FOR LITHIUM

I usually initiate treatment with **Eskalith 300 mg**(#15) two or three times daily. The clinical history helps me decide only approximately if they have healthy kidneys. If test doses of lithium work, they are prescribed more and are to use 900 mg or less per day for a week, at which time they obtain baseline labs:

Initial and Annual Labs

- **Thyroid profile with TSH**
- **Electrolytes, BUN, Creatinine**
- UA, and lithium level
- CBC, calcium level
- Thyroid antibodies: anti-thyroglobulin, antimitochondrial
- Electrocardiogram if over 40

This is drawn 12 hours after the last lithium dose, 7 days after a steady amount has been taken. An ECG is ordered, especially if heart disease is suspected. Standard psychiatry recommends all of the above labs **before** lithium is started.

For patients well enough to not be in a hospital, I often prefer flexible brief medication trials occur before cumbersome, expensive bloodwork. As soon as a decision is made to continue a medication, then normal lab testing can be done. Due to this delay for physically healthy appearing outpatients, I caution them to discontinue lithium if **toxic signs** are occurring (severe nausea, vomiting, diarrhea, staggering, confusion). I recognize this is not ideal. Yet it frees up a large population to quickly assess lithium or some other protocol medication when lab work isn't in the way. In my nine years of work there has not been a problem with this approach. Perhaps this is because protocol doses are very low and brief.

139

The risk of kidney injury due to long term lithium treatment is lower than formally believed. In one study, kidney function remained stable for 20 years. Problems arise when lithium intoxication occurs (overdosing), or when the kidneys were already diseased before treatment started. Being careful about keeping the lithium level as low as possible, and taking adequate fluids throughout the day I believe should protect the kidneys.

A Lithium level in the range of 0.3-1 is often excellent. Standard psychiatry recommends 0.6-.8 as maintenance, and 0.8-1 as very therapeutic. Usually people show toxic signs by 1.2, and the elderly by half that level, so it is safer to keep well below this.

Standard psychiatry recommends lithium levels should be checked at least twice weekly initially, weekly after dosage changes, then every 3 months. Levels are ordered more often if fever, vomiting, diarrhea, dehydration or weight loss are occurring. If lithium is being started and given in a lower dose range, I am more relaxed concerning the **blood monitoring**. Thus in this situation, a blood lithium level I order initially after the lithium is working and semi-annually thereafter (or more often if dosage is raised or toxic signs occur). If the lithium level is rising when all other factors are constant, that may be the earliest sign of a lithium related change in kidney function. That is why it is important to be consistent about when the lithium level is drawn (i.e., each time 12 hours after the prior dose).

In up to 30%, lithium may worsen or cause a **hypothyroid change**. Blood work (thyroid profile with TSH, perhaps thyroid antibodies) should be checked any time hypothyroid clinical signs are occurring (page 47). This may show a confirmatory rising TSH.

If lithium tremor occurs, it often disappears after 2-3 weeks of treatment. The lithium dose may however be lowered or **Inderal** may be added.

Inderal 20mg: 1/2-1 tablet 3-4 times per day

Pregnant women should not be started on lithium.

DEPAKOTE

DEPAKOTE DESTABILIZATION

Patients may feel worse, moody, tense, agitated, get a headache or become very sedated at a normal dose. The medication may initially work, then stop working. Sometimes these are just side effects, but more often signify a different underlying chemistry is present.

MEDICAL EFFECTS

Too much Depakote can cause nausea and sedation. More often the medicine is slightly activating.

Patients with liver disease should not take Depakote. These people and children under 2 years of age, can potentially die from liver toxicity while taking the medicine.

Menstrual changes can occur in 20%. Other side effects occur 5% (or less frequently) and include upset stomach, diarrhea, salivation, easy bruising, rashes, hair loss, weakness, headache, and sedation. (Reference 20, page 166.)

140

LAB WORK FOR DEPAKOTE

Depakote is hazardous if liver disease or failure is occurring. If a patient does not have jaundiced eyes, I believe the liver profile labs can wait, indefinitely until blood is drawn for any other reason. Yet a liver damaged alcoholic or someone with hepatitis should be monitored. Dosage can be raised above 250mg three times a day, to 1250 mg/day. Blood level can be 50-120ug/ml. With Depakote, I rarely use high doses, or get blood levels. If a medicine is showing signs of working at a moderate level, it may be worth increasing the dose and checking blood levels if toxicity, or interaction with other medications is a concern.

TEGRETAL

Tegretal structurally resembles Pamelar and, so like the antidepressants, can induce bipolar destabilization at a rate of 12%.

TEGRETAL DESTABILIZATION

Patients may feel worse, uneasy, agitated, stressed, fidgety, confused, volatile, weak, "zombied", like their skin is "crawling", sweaty or uncoordinated at a normal dose. This can destabilize like an antidepressant. The medication may initially work, then stop working. Sometimes these are just side effects, but more often signify a different underlying chemistry is present.

MEDICAL EFFECTS OF TEGRETAL

Symptoms: Too much Tegretal can cause **nausea, sedation,** dizziness, confusion, and poor coordination (with speech, vision, and walking). Vision can be blurred and double. Dosage is determined clinically, and not with blood levels.

Blood Count: Mild reversible changes can occur in the blood; Up to a 25% reduction in **WBC COUNT** in 11%, (and elevated **liver functions**): In 2% the **lowered WBC** count (less than 3000WBC/mm^3) or thrombocyte count can persist. 5% bruise easily. **Mild anemia** can occur in less than 5% of patients. Bone marrow suppression effects 3% and can include rare agranulocytosis, pancytopenia, eosinophilia, purpura. Rare **aplastic anemia** or agranulocytosis occurs once in every 100,000 patients. Most patients using Tegretal for moods require a low dose of 200-300 mg per day.

Stop Tegretal If

- WBC count is less than 3,000/mm^3.
- Neutrophil count is less than 1500.
- Liver function tests elevated 3-fold.
- Fever and rash in first month.
- Easy bruising, pinpoint red spots on skin.

Heart: Blood pressure can be lowered (dizziness) or elevated and **conduction** times (atrioventricular) in the heart can be decreased. Thus if a patient has a heart block, Tegretal should be used carefully.

Stomach: If nausea, indigestion or vomiting occur, take the medicine with food, and lower the dose.

Kidney: Urinary frequency rarely can occur (inappropriate ADH secretion). Dry mouth and water intoxication confusion can occur.

Skin Allergies: Rashes are common (7%) with Tegretal, usually within the 2nd and 3rd week of treatment. (Reference 20)

      A. Allergic

      B. Scaling loss of skin layers

      C. Erosive lesions in mucosal areas (mouth) with effects on eyes.

Hay fever, shortness of breath, pneumonitis, and pneumonia can occur.

Fever, enlarged lymph nodes, joint aches, chills, and sweating can also occur.

A rare, occasionally fatal reaction with fever and rash can occur during the first month. (I have never seen this.)

Neurologic: Confusion and agitation can occur when combining Tegretal with other mood stabilizers, particularly lithium, or neuroleptics. - 12% have mania induced with Tegretal. (Reference 20)

LAB WORK FOR TEGRETAL

The lab test **"CBC with reticulocyte count"** is ordered if they like the medicine. The blood level for epilepsy control should be 6-12 ug/ml, but effective doses for psychiatric disorders usually result from doses of 100 mg, 2-3 times a day, so I rarely check the blood level.

Just as sun can be toxic on the skin, tegretol can be toxic on the bone marrow. A full dose of Tegretol is 1200 mg/day, so the low 200-300 mg per day dose range helps to avoid trouble. If dosage needs raised, this can be done. Most people find higher doses too sedating, or nauseating. **Quarterly** CBC blood tests are recommended, and can also be done twice monthly the first two months to watch out for a persistent decrease in WBC's which could signal aplastic anemia, which occurs less than once every 100,000 patients. If the WBC count falls to 4,000 mm³, repeat the CBC in 2 weeks. If the test is still abnormal, reduce Tegretal.

Lab: CBC with reticulocyte count

British experts believe the blood tests are unnecessary unless one sees signs of bone marrow suppression such as fever, sore throat and pinpoint red spots on the skin (Reference 14, page 170).

KLONOPIN - MEDICATION TOXICITY

This medicine stabilizes seizures (electricity) similar to Depakote, but also has practically identical structure to Ativan, a benzodiazepine. See the section on benzodiazepines for medical effects.

ANTIPSYCHOTIC DESTABILIZATION

A patient taking antipsychotic may feel worse, confused, agitated, irritable, "wired", or have nightmares. Often these are just side effects (Akathisia - page 144). Yet sometimes these symptoms signify that there is no dopamine elevation, and that a different underlying chemistry is present.

MEDICAL EFFECTS OF ANTIPSYCHOTICS ("NEUROLEPTICS") *see graph on page 70*

Anticholinergic: These usually decrease in 1-2 weeks: **Dry mouth**, constipation (gut can be temporarily paralyzed), urinary hesitancy/retention, **low blood pressure,** dry eyes, blurred vision, narrow-angle glaucoma, light sensitivity, nasal congestion, drying of throat and breathing. R_x - Switch to a different less problematic antipsychotic by choosing from the graph on page 70.

Heart: Low Blood Pressure, if serious can be treated with metaraminol, phenylephrine or norepinephrine, but not epinephrine. Legs can be elevated and head lowered until a different antipsychotic is chosen from the graph.

Digestive: Dry mouth can be improved by changing medicines, or adding a saliva substitute Xero-Lube, or pilocarpine 1% solution (mouth wash) or a bethanechol 5-10mg tablet dissolved in water (cholinergic mouth wash).

Constipation may respond to switching medicines (a less anticholinergic antipsychotic), or to increasing dietary bulk (bran, metamucil), or stool softener (docusate), or bethanechol 10-25mg, 3-4 times per day, or in an emergency, giving a laxative. Allergic obstructive <u>hepatitis</u> used to occur primarily after chlorpromazine (thorazine) was introduced, less than once every thousand patients. Yellowing of the eyes, and hepatitis, cleared by stopping the medicine.

Weight gain can frequently be turned into weight loss by using molindone (Moban), yet neurotoxic reactions (confusion, distress) occur more often with this medicine in my practice.

Kidneys: Urinary hesitancy can contribute to more urinary tract infections. A less anticholinergic antipsychotic should be chosen. R_x - Bethanechol 10-25mg, 3-4 times a day or 5-10mg hourly until better. Bethanechol can be given IM or subcutaneously (5-10mg) if necessary.

Endocrine: Breasts in 0-2%, can enlarge, be tender, and rarely secrete milk drops. **Sex drive** and orgasm may be diminished in 25%.

Menstrual irregularities can occur. Thioridazine (Mellaril), which is good in many ways, has the worst statistics sexually; ejaculation can even be backwards into the bladder. Sustained erection can very rarely occur with some antipsychotics which lower blood pressure the most (see graph on page 70).

Blood sugar changes (low or high) can also occur, and produce sugar in the urine.

Blood: Agranulocytosis is when the WBC count drops to less than $1,000-2,000/mm^3$, with neutrophils less than $500/mm^3$. This occurs in fewer than **one in 5,000** patients, and mostly with clozapine (Clozaril) - 1.3%, or chlorpromazine (Thorazine) - 0.7%. The onset can be sudden, during the first 3 months, and usually is in the first month of treatment.

If **sore throat, high fever** and perhaps **mouth ulcers** or sores occur, stop antipsychotics. A person can die if the medicine is not stopped. Other signs can include stomach distress, weakness, enlarged lymph nodes, asthma, skin ulcers, fluid retention, and severe allergic reactions ("anaphylactic"). If a patient has less than a $3,000-3,500/mm^3$ WBC count, do not start antipsychotic medication. Frequent blood work helps only for Clozaril.

Leukopenia is a milder form of agranulocytosis where WBC count is reduced to $2,000-3,500/mm^3$. Symptoms are similar, and antipsychotic should be stopped or reduced.

Eyes: Blurring may be fixed by picking a less anticholinergic neuroleptic. Otherwise prescribe pilocarpine 1% eye drops, one drop 3 times per day, (1 or 15ml containers), or bethanechol 5-10mg, 3 to 4 times per day.

Eye pigmentation (in back of cornea and front of the lens) can occur in 6% of patients taking

Thorazine, Navane or Taractin after long term use; the pupil looks opaque if a light is shined into it. Skin pigmentation can also occur. With extreme doses of Mellaril (thioridazine) in excess of 800mg per day, for more than several days, the retina (back of eye) can become pigmented causing decreased vision or blindness.

Narrow angle glaucoma can occur with the most anticholinergic neuroleptics (see page 70). Symptoms include pain in the eye or face, blurring and sometimes halos being seen around lights.

Skin: **Sunburn** can occur more quickly while taking antipsychotics. Also **temperature instability** can rarely occur. Most often a patient can feel too cool, but overheating with decreased sweating is more dangerous.

Neurologic: Easily correctable side effects, called EPS (extrapyramidal symptoms), occur in about 50% of patients. They are preventable by prescribing a side effect pill with the neuroleptic, or using the lowest effective dose of neuroleptic.

Muscle cramps - (**"Dystonia"**) in Jaw, Tongue, Neck or back

- R_x: Cogentin 1-2 mg 2-3 times per day.
- or R_x: Benadryl 25-50 mg 3-4 times per day.

Either can be given as a shot (IV/IM) in the above doses.
Note: Benadryl can be bought over the counter at grocery stores. A 12.5mg dose often works and is less sedating.

Restless (**"Akathisia"**)
Uncomfortable
Anxious
Fidgety

- R_x: Artane 2-5 mg 2-3 times per day
- or R_x: Inderal 10-20 mg 2-3 times per day.

Shuffling, (**"Pseudo Parkinsons"**)
Weak, Slowed, or (**"Akinesia"**)
Apathetic,
Stiff,
Reduced Movement,
Drooling

- R_x: Cogentin 0.5-1 mg 2-3 times per day.
- or R_x: Artane 2 mg 2-3 times per day
- or R_x: Amantadine 100mg 1/2 -1 tablet 2-3 times per day for the **Elderly**.

Rapid Lip (**"Rabbit Syndrome"**)
Tremor

- R_x: Artane 2-5 mg 2-3 times per day
- or R_x: Cogentin 0.5-1 mg 2-3 times per day.

More serious side effects include the following two problems:

1. TARDIVE DYSKINESIA

According to the literature, in about 20-25% of patients, potentially irreversible tardive dyskinesia side effects can occur, usually after more than two years of high dose neuroleptic treatment. My experience is I have never seen this in low dose treatment.

TARDIVE DYSKINESIA SYMPTOMS (Can Include)

Face   **Chewing**, **smacking**, grimacing, puckering, rolling the tongue, frowning, smiling, licking, blinking, etc.

Limbs   Snake-like movements, tremors, foot tapping, squirming, twisting.

Body   Rocking, squirming, twisting, thrusting, jerking.

They **usually go away if the neuroleptic is stopped** or switched to a less potent neuroleptic class.

MEDICATIONS WHICH MIGHT INHIBIT TARDIVE DYSKINESIA INCLUDE:

Amantadine 100mg: 2-3 times per day.

Baclofen 5-20mg: 3 times per day.

Benzodiazepines (Librium, Valium).

Carbamazepine 100mg: 1-2 tablets 3 times per day.

Choline 2-8 grams per day.

Clonidine 0.3-0.7mg per day.

Lecithin 10-40 grams per day.

Levodopa 100-2000mg per day.

Lithium 300mg: 3 times per day.

Reserpine 1-6mg per day.

Valproic Acid 1000-1500mg per day.

Vitamin E.

2. NEUROLEPTIC MALIGNANT SYNDROME

In about 2% of the patients, a dangerous side effect, **Neuroleptic Malignant Syndrome** can kill 18% of victims according to the literature. In my experience, it has always been reversible.

NEUROLEPTIC MALIGNANT SYNDROME Can Include

Severe pseudo-Parkinsons (see page 144).
Fever (101-107^0).
Dazed, confused, almost mute, agitated, incontinent, in a stupor.
Increased heart rate, blood pressure, breathing.
Sweating, salivating, poor swallowing.
Lab Work Shows: Increased white blood cell count(15,000-30,000/mm^3).
                              Increased creatinine phosphate (347 to 4,286 u/ml).
                              Elevated liver function tests.
                              Myoglobinuria, renal failure.
*This condition definitely occurs and should be watched out for.

The typical cause is a rapidly increasing **high neuroleptic dose**. 67% were taking a **high potency** neuroleptic. Some were taking 2 or more antipsychotics. When Neuroleptic Malignant Syndrome occurs, most fatalities have happened with:

trifluoperazine (Stelazine)	43%
chlorpromazine (Thorazine)	40%
thiothixene (Navane)	40%
fluphenazine shot (Prolixin)	33%

Much <u>fewer fatalities</u> occur with:

thioridazine (**Mellaril**)	0%
haloperidol (**Haldol**)	5.5%
fluphenazine tablets (**Prolixin**)	8.3%

NMS TREATMENT

• Early identification.
• Stop all antipsychotics (and anticholinergics).
• Maintain good hydration (oral or I.V.)
• **Bromocriptine** 5 mg every 4 hours to relieve rigidity and fever. (Range
   7.5-60 mg per day)
• Cool body if feverish.
• Avoid antipsychotics for 1 month, then cautiously restart Mellaril.

Dantroline 2-3 mg/kg per day has been used for NMS instead of bromocriptine, but reports are not as favorable.

STIMULANT DESTABILIZATION

A patient taking stimulant may feel worse, moody, irritable, volatile, confused, agitated, destructive, sad, or "speedy". Palpitations, hallucinations or severe insomnia can occur. If the medicine initially worked, neuroleptic may need to be added, or the stimulant may need to be switched to a different one. The above destabilization signs can be side effects or signify that a different underlying chemistry is present.

MEDICAL EFFECTS

In treating ADD chemistry, stimulants do not induce physical dependence, tolerance or addiction. Contraindications: hypertensive, cardiovasular and hyperthyroid patients should not have stimulant.

Heart: Dizziness can occur in 12% on Dexedrine, 8% on Ritalin, and 6% on Cylert.
 Higher blood pressure can occur in 10% on Dexedrine and 16% on Ritalin.
 Rapid heart rate can occur in 6% on Dexedrine and Cylert, but 15% on Ritalin.
 Palpitations occurs in about 5%.
 Heart irregularity or chest pain can occur in less than 1% on Dexedrine, but in about 5% on Ritalin.

Digestive: Dry mouth can occur in about 9%
 Lower appetite occurs in 30% of children on high stimulant doses.
 Nausea occurs in about 5%.
 Abdominal pain can also happen.
 Weight loss occurs in 30% on Dexedrine, 14% on Ritalin and 5% on Cylert. All these stomach problems may clear in 2-6 weeks, with treatment continuing. Otherwise, switching to a gentler stimulant can help. Ritalin causes weight gain in 4%,and Cylert can cause gain after 3-6 months.
 Growth suppression is most with Dexedrine, then Ritalin, and least with Cylert. Full growth rebound occurs when the medicine is stopped, i.e. during school vacations each summer, or during adolescence when the medicine is discontinued. Some sources say growth can only temporarily be suppressed by any stimulant.

Liver toxicity can occur with Cylert. Enzymes (SGOT and SGPT) become reversibly elevated. There are rare reports of fatality. Symptoms include, after several months, fatigue and stomach fullness.

Bladder: Bed-wetting can occur in 9% on Ritalin.

Skin/Allergies: Rashes, hives, **joint pains,** or **fever** can occur in 6% on Ritalin. Dexedrine can cause **sweating** in 6%.

Neurologic: Insomnia occurs in 19% on Dexedrine, 17% on Ritalin, and 29% on Cylert (often normalizes). Giving doses earlier in the day, or switching to a shorter acting, perhaps weaker stimulant can help.
 Sedation and drowsiness occurs in 6%. Difficulty in waking occurs in 15% on Ritalin.
 Confusion occurs in 10% on Dexedrine, and 4% on Ritalin.
 Irritability occurs in 25% on Dexedrine, 17% on Ritalin, and 13% on Cylert.
 Depression occurs in 39% on Dexedrine, and 9% on Ritalin.
 A **mood change** of mild sadness, withdrawal, dulled emotions and overconcentrating occurs in 10% with Ritalin and less than 1% with Dexedrine.
 Psychosis is induced in less than 1%. This clears by lowering stimulant dose, switching to milder

stimulant or adding neuroleptic. An emergency dose of Stelazine 1-2mg usually provides relief, until other adjustments are made.

Headache occurs in 18% on Dexedrine, 9% on Ritalin, and 14% on Cylert.

Tremor occurs in 6% with Ritalin or Dexedrine.

Motor tics (squints, grimaces) can occur in less than 1%. Underlying tourettes should be considered. Options include using Clonidine, switching to a milder stimulant, stopping the stimulant, or treating tourettes if that is the true primary diagnosis. Neuroleptic and stimulant can be combined if necessary.

Seizures have been reported from Cylert, but not with Ritalin, Dexedrine or Ionamin. Tenuate (similar in structure to Wellbutrin) also has an increased rate of seizures in epileptics. All in overdose can cause seizures.

Withdrawal symptoms can occur when stimulant is abused chronically, then stopped. The person has increased sleep, fatigue and appetite for one to several days. Depression or paranoia can also occur.

LAB WORK FOR STIMULANT

Cylert can be monitored with periodic blood tests (liver functions) to guard against rare hepatic toxicity.

For **Ritalin**, periodic CBC, differential and platelet counts are recommended during long term treatment due to rare blood disturbances (anemia, bruising) which can be induced.

BENZODIAZEPINE DESTABILIZATION

Sometimes patients taking this can feel much worse, depressed, labile, moody, agitated or distressed. One variety of benzodiazepine might cause this while others do not. This may be a side effect, but usually reflects different underlying chemistry is present.

MEDICAL EFFECTS - BENZODIAZEPINES FOR ANXIETY

Heart: Mild **dizziness** and lightheadness can occur in 13%.
> **Palpitations** can happen in 7%.

Digestive: Dry mouth occurs in 13% and **nausea, diarrhea,** or **constipation** occur in 7%.

Allergies: Rash or **itching** occurs in 6%.

Neurologic:
> **blurred vision** occurs in 11%.
> **sexual** functioning is disturbed in 11%.
> **Headache** happens in 9%.
> **Drowsiness** occurs in 35%,
> **clumsiness** in 20%, and
> **incoordination** or **weakness** in 18%.
> **Depression** occurs in 8%.
> **Disorientation** in 7%,
> **insomnia** in 6%,
> **hostility** in 6%,
> **hallucinations** in 5% and
> **anxiety** in 4%.

BENZODIAZEPINES FOR SLEEP

Hangover drowsiness tends to be worse with medications that have a long half life (Dalmane 74 hrs.).

Falls can occur from dizziness in 1.5% on Doral, 11% on Halcion, 13% on Restoril, and 24% on Dalmane.

Patients with **respiratory problems** (for example asthma, chronic obstructive pulmonary disease) should not take sleep medicines.

Amnesia has occurred with Halcion for events occurring up to 11 hours after taking the medicine.

Tolerance can occur over several months. Halcion can often simply be stopped and restarted in a day or two.

ADDICTION TO BENZODIAZEPINES

Many patients need this type of medication and do not appear to grow tolerant.
Others show signs of dependence and gradually escalating dose requirement. The most major risk of benzodiazepine treatment concerns impaired judgement and coordination leading to car accidents. Nevertheless, what follows are approximate rates of addiction at different dose levels (Reference 9, page 528).

BENZODIAZEPINE	DOSE PER DAY	TIME FRAME TO BECOME ADDICTED
Xanax	1.5-3.0 mg	3-11 months
Librium	300-600 mg	2-6 months
Valium	15-30 mg	several years
	80 mg or more	6 weeks
Ativan	8 mg	6 months
	12mg or more	6 weeks
Serax	30-60 mg	1 year
Dalmane	60-90 mg	several months
Halcion	0.5-5.0 mg	2-3 months
Chloral hydrate	2,000 mg	several months
Phenobarbital	200 mg	several years

Standard psychiatry may be over utilizing benzodiazepines when other access points could have more efficiently and safely solved the problem. There is a minority that do well primarily with benzodiazepine GABA enhancement treatment. If someone becomes addicted, it is usually a simple matter to apply protocol 1-3 to locate a safer more effective approach.

WITHDRAWAL FROM BENZODIAZEPINES

If these medicines are abruptly stopped after being taken several months in high dose, dangerous withdrawal can occur. Symptoms can include anxiety, tremor, sweating, agitation, abdominal or muscle cramping, vomiting, disorientation, seizures and death.

Mild discomfort can follow discontinuation of a lower dose benzodiazepine. It is important to taper these medications slowly and gently "as tolerated" when you want to stop them.

CYTOMEL,	SYNTHROID,
TRIOSTAT (IV),	ARMOUR,
LEVOTHROID,	S-P-T
LEVOXYL,	THYRAR
	THYROLAR

THYROID MEDICATION DESTABILIZATION

A patient taking thyroid may feel worse, agitated, anxious, confused, insomnic, disorganized, disoriented, or hyperactive. They may be taking excessive thyroid, or have a different underlying chemical imbalance.

MEDICAL EFFECTS OF THYROID MEDICINE

Cardiovascular: Use thyroid hormone with great caution if coronary artery disease (especially in the elderly) or angina are present. Rapid heart rate, palpitations and angina can occur.

Endocrine: In women, TSH suppression by thyroid medicines to very low or undetectable levels may increase bone resorption, **osteoporosis** and risk of bone fracture. Thus it is recommended by the American Medical Association to limit thyroid dosage to amounts that reduce serum TSH to a low normal range.

Diabetes and Addisons disease can be worsened with thyroid hormone.

Blood: Patients who require anticoagulant may have longer clotting times as thyroid is increased.

LAB WORK FOR THYROID

The hypothyroid checklist is often sensitive as an indicator of thyroid malfunction (see page 47). Lab tests are occasionally confirmatory. An elevated **TSH,** and sometimes decreased **Free T**$_4$ are the accepted standard for defining hypothyroidism. The **FTI** (free thyroxine index) is useful. **Anti-T** and **Anti-M** antibodies (antithyroglobulin, antimicrosomal) indicate autoimmune thyroid disease and are sometimes positive in symptomatic patients when all other thyroid tests are normal. Other autoimmune antibody tests can be ordered (see page 112).

If **Synthroid** (T$_4$) is given, progress can be monitored by improvement in symptoms, and normalization of the Free T$_4$, FTI, and TSH. Synthroid closely matches the physiologic needs of hypothyroid victims and offers more gentle consistency.

If **Cytomel** (T$_3$) is given, progress can be monitored by symptom decrease, and lowering of the TSH to a low normal range. This medicine may be more stimulating for thyroid resistant patients and those who don't metabolize T$_4$ to T$_3$. Cytomel is shorter acting and has T$_3$ in a quantity 5 times the physiologic ratio of T$_3$ to T$_4$. Since Cytomel does not replace T$_4$, the Free T$_4$ and FTI are not reliable indexes, but the TSH is.

Mixed preparations are considered to offer no advantage.

Estrogen often helps hot flashes, vaginal inflammation/dryness, urinary urgency/incontinence, and sometimes mental symptoms. Estrogen can cause fluid retention, nausea, uterine bleeding, breast tenderness, uterine fibroid increase in size, areas of skin pigmentation and high calcium levels if bone disease or bone metastasis is present.

Bone mineral loss (osteoporosis) is reduced to the degree that hip fractures occur 25% less. Bone mass can be assessed.
Coronary heart disease is reduced 35-50%.

Yet, estrogen alone can increase uterine endometrial cancer risk. Besides having a low fatality rate, this risk appears to be eliminated by progestins being given a minimum of 10-12 days per month (reference 8).

Post menopausal estrogen use causes a 30% increased risk of **breast cancer.** Thus, women with a family history of this may prefer no estrogen treatments. However, estrogen's therapeutic reduction in heart disease far outweighs the risk of cancer. Thus postmenopausal women without contraindications should consider this hormonal treatment.

CONTRAINDICATIONS TO ESTROGEN Rx

Breast Cancer
Estrogen dependent cancer (breast, endometrial, melanoma, liver
      hepatoma / hepatocellular)
Thromboembolic disorders (blood clots, stroke)
Genital bleeding of unknown cause
Pregnancy
Liver disease (active)

POSSIBLE CONTRAINDICATIONS

Mild liver disease
Past blood clots
Gallbladder disease
Uterine fibroids
Endometriosis
Migraine
Epilepsy
Hypertension
Porphyria
Familial hyperlipidemia

ESTROGEN LAB WORK: Serum Estrogen, FSH, LH

CHAPTER 10

OVERDOSES

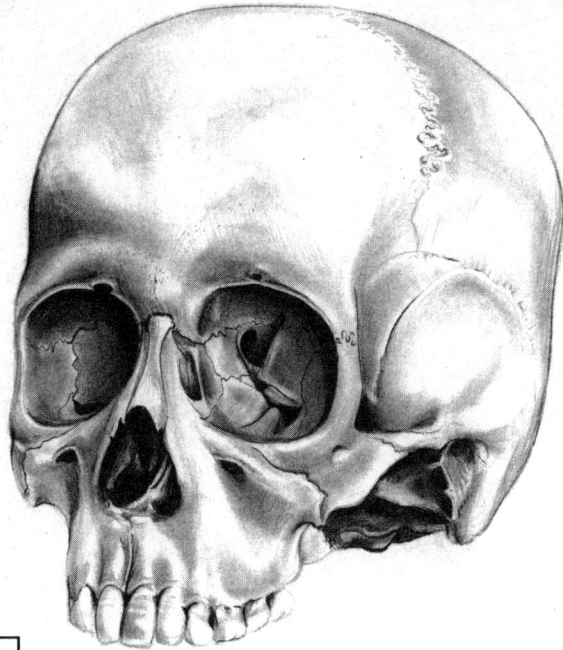

SUICIDALITY

If a suicide attempt is about to occur, <u>Stelazine 2mg</u> can be held in the mouth on the tongue until feelings are better (1-2 minutes). The medicine is then swallowed. If the Stelazine can be cut or broken, it is absorbed faster. <u>Xanax</u> 0.5mg can be swallowed for additional comfort. *Patients should contact their doctor immediately or go to an emergency room.*

Overdose Treatments were Reviewed by: Los Angeles Regional Drug and Poison Information Center, Margaret McCarron MD, FACP Medicine/Emergency Medicine USC

OVERDOSE: GENERAL PRINCIPALS OF TREATMENT

Emesis (vomiting): This is the most effective way to empty the stomach. Yet if the person is too drowsy or unconscious, this should not be done since they could choke on their vomit.

Syrup of Ipecac
> Contraindicated in children under 6 months of age.
> 6 to 12 months: 5 to 10ml followed by 10-20ml/Kg of water
> 1 to 12 years: 15ml followed by 10-20ml/kg of water
> Older children, adults: 30ml followed by 200-300ml of water
> Dosage may be repeated one time if vomiting does not occur in *20 minutes.*

> Syrup of ipecac is rarely used in emergency departments today, but is administered at home after calling the local Poison Center to see if syrup of ipecac is contraindicated for the substance taken.

Absorption:
> For most drug overdoses, **Activated Charcoal Suspension** in water is the preferred treatment. However, this is not a satisfactory treatment for small children at home, since children do not like the taste, won't take it, or spit it up over parent, wall, etc.

> For adult patients in emergency departments, activated charcoal solution is either given alone or as part of the gastric lavage:

> > Dangerous if drowsy, be sure to use cuffed endotracheal intubation.

> Ewald tube is inserted (prior endotracheal intubation may be required in some cases) with patient sitting or with the head of the bed raised.

> Contents of stomach are aspirated and examined visually.

> Activated charcoal suspension (80 to 100 grams) is instilled in the stomach to bind with the toxin before lavaging with water—to prevent solubilizing of the toxin and increasing its absorption.

> Tap water lavage is done until return solution is clear.

> Activated charcoal suspension, or activated charcoal in Sorbitol if a cathartic is desired, dose 60-80 grams, is instilled in the stomach.

> Ewald tube is removed.

> **For children: Activated charcoal suspension single oral doses:**

> Infants less than 1 year old: 1 gm/Kg of body weight

> 1 to 12 years old: 1 to 2 gm/Kg of 15 to 30 gm.

> Overdoses with seizure risk usually should not have vomiting induced.

> Supportive Measures: Victims need close observation.

Seizures can be treated with

Diazepam (Valium) 5-10mg IV given over 2-3 minutes

or Lorazepam (Ativan) 2-3mg IV.

If seizures continue: Phenobarbital 15-20mg/kg IV and/or Phenytoin 15mg/kg IV is given over 30 or more minutes.

The room can be darkened to minimize stimulation that could induce a seizure (especially from strychnine poisoning).

ANTIDEPRESSANT OVERDOSES

SNRI, SSRI OVERDOSE

Newer antidepressants (Effexor, Luvox, Paxil, Prozac, Zoloft) are not as toxic to the heart, and are safer. Overdoses combined with other drugs can cause severe toxicity.

TREATMENT

The mainstay of treatment is **close observation**, and **symptomatic supportive care**, with cardiac monitoring. Maintain an airway and ventilation . For an adult give 60-80 grams of activated charcoal suspension every 4-6 hours for 24-48 hours after the overdose (if paralytic ileus is not present). Dialysis, forced diuresis and hemoperfusion are unlikely to help.

Effexor Overdoses up to 6,750mg caused somnolence, and usually no symptoms. One patient however had seizures and cardiac conduction changes. Rapid heart rate occasionally occurred.

Paxil - No deaths reported (from overdoses up to 850mg). Symptoms include nausea, vomiting, drowsiness, rapid heart rate and dilated pupils.

Zoloft - Overdoses up to 2100mg have not resulted in serious symptoms. No deaths reported (from overdoses up to 6000mg). There is a recommendation to add charcoal in sorbitol to evacuate the bowels if multiple dose charcoal therapy is not being done.

Prozac - Overdoses up to 800mg seem to cause minimal toxicity. Nausea, vomiting, seizures, sedation and coma can occur with overdoses. Several deaths have occurred when Prozac was mixed with other medicines in overdose. At twice the maximum human dose, seizures can be induced in dogs. Treatment is the same as for Zoloft, except for needing to be prepared to treat seizures (see Tricyclic section).
Cardiac monitoring should be done.

Luvox - Overdoses can result in death, but usually this is when mixed with other drugs. 87% have complete recovery after gastric lavage. Activated charcoal may be as effective as emesis or lavage. Drowsiness, vomiting, diarrhea and dizziness occur; seizures and ECG abnormalities are possible.

Anafranil, Ascendin, Desyrel, Elavil, Ludiomil, Norpramine, Pamelar, Serzone, Sinequan, Surmontil, Tofranil, Wellbutrin, Vivactil

Tricyclic antidepressants are often fatal at 30-40mg/kg in adults, and 20mg/kg in children. Severe toxicity is seen at 10-20mg/kg in adults. TCA's are highly tissue-bound and are not removed effectively by hemodialysis, peritoneal dialysis, exchange transfusions or forced diuresis. Overdose symptoms may start in 30-60 minutes.

Anticholinergic effects include delirium, dilated pupils, rapid heart rate, dry mouth, flushed skin (less sweating), fever, hypertension, muscle twitches, constipation, and urinary retention.

Heart depressant effects include **QRS interval widening** to greater than 0.12 seconds (if below 0.10, ventricular arrhythmias are less frequent), QT interval to more than 441 msec, QTc of 500 msec or more, ventricular arrhythmias, atrioventricular block, and low blood pressure.

Seizures and **coma** are common with serious overdoses. Hyperthermia can result from seizures and lack of sweating. After clothes are removed, the patient can be sprayed with water and fanned. Ice packs can be used. If temperature is 105F or more rectally, ice water lavage and ice water enemas can be done.

Treatment

Maintain the **airway**, assist ventilation if necessary. If the **ECG** is abnormal, do continuous cardiac monitoring. Perform gastric **lavage** and administer activated **charcoal** suspension. Do not induce vomiting as this can induce seizures. A cuffed endotracheal tube can be placed before lavage in groggy or unconscious patients. If the patient has ileus, which is very common, the sorbitol will remain in the GI tract and cause distension with fluid accumulation; if the pressure in the lumen of the bowel increases it can cause ischemic necrosis of the bowel lining and death. This will not happen with activated charcoal in water suspension.

Bowel sounds should also be monitored, and the stomach should be **aspirated before the next activated charcoal suspension dose is given**. If charcoal is recovered from the stomach four hours after it was instilled, the **stomach is atonic** and no further charcoal should be given. Overdistending the stomach can lead to vomiting and aspiration of charcoal into the lungs. Heart depression may respond to boluses of **sodium bicarbonate** (50-100meg IV, or 1-2meg/kg). PH should be maintained at 7.5 (acidosis is usually severe) for at least 24 hours.

Ventricular arrhythmias can be treated with Phenytoin, Lidocaine, or Propranolol. Avoid quinidine, procainamide, disopyramide, which can worsen TCA arrhythmias.

Shock can be treated by positioning, IV fluids and if necessary, pressor agents.

Seizures can be treated with Diazepam (Valium) 5-10mg IV given over 2-3minutes or Lorazepam (Ativan) 2-3mg IV.

If seizures continue: Phenobarbital 15-20mg/kg IV and/or Phenytoin 15mg/kg IV is given over 30 or more minutes.

The room can be darkened to minimize stimulation that could induce a seizure. Due to urinary retention, a **urinary catheter** may be inserted to help the patient void, if necessary.

Nardil, Parnate

The highest toxic doses of Nardil or Parnate are 750mg, with fatality occurring usually at 1,000mg, but as low as 375mg. Early symptoms include staggering, dizziness, excitement, irritability, headache, drowsiness, rigid arching hyperextension of the body, lockjaw, **hypertension** and rapid irregular heart rate. Symptoms may maximize at 24-48 hours, and can include **hypotension**, shock, cardiovascular insufficiency, myocardial infarction, and arrhythmias. **Seizures**, **hyperthermia**, confusion, hallucinations, rigidity, muscle spasms, respiratory depression, and coma can occur. If tyramine-containing foods are eaten, or sympathomimetic drugs are taken, severe hypertensive reactions can occur. Meperidine (Demerol), Prozac or other SSRI's with MAOI, can cause fatal fever. Symptoms usually clear in 3-4 days, but can continue 2 weeks.

Treatment

Follow MAOI dietary and drug restrictions carefully. Give activated charcoal in sorbitol after lavage is completed. Severe **hypertension** (diastolic greater than 105-110mm Hg) is treated with: Nitroprusside sodium, 0.25-8ug/kg/min IV or - Phentolamine 2-5mg IV. If rapid heart rate is present, propranolol 1-5mg IV, or esmolol 25-100ug/kg/min IV can be added, but not given alone (can worsen hypertension). For **hypotension**, push fluids and avoid administering pressor amines such as norepinephrine. **Seizures** can be treated as in the TCA section. External cooling can help **hyperthermia**. Liver function tests should be done in about 4-6 weeks to monitor for liver toxicity.

LITHIUM OVERDOSE

There are two types of lithium intoxication: acute and chronic. Chronic lithium overdose occurs from too high daily dosage, decreased fluid intake, or a change in the water balance. An overdose can cause **permanent injury** in 10% and may be characterized by confusion, dementia, staggering, frequent urination, speech difficulties, spasticity, tremor, heart irregularity, falling blood pressure, and seizures. **Death** occurs in 10-25% and usually at doses of 10,000-60,000mg.

Treatment

Labs - ECG, lithium level, electrolytes, creatinine, glucose, and urinalysis. **Gastric Lavage, Correction of fluid and electrolyte imbalance:** 0.9% IV sodium chloride (1-2 liters within 6 hours) for low sodium. **Hemodialysis** immediately for 8-12 hours is indicated if the lithium level is 3meg/l or more, or if the patient is worsening with a level of 2meg/l or greater. Hemodialysis is indicated again eight hours after the last hemodialysis, if fluid or electrolyte abnormalities do not respond, if creatinine clearance or urine output decrease markedly, or if the lithium level is not less than 1meg/l. Seizures are treated with short acting barbiturates such as Thiopental. Lithium can be restarted 48 hours after the patient is medically well.

DEPAKOTE OVERDOSE

An overdose can cause nausea, vomiting, lethargy, staggering, tremor, heart block, deep coma, and fatality. Liver toxicity can occur in children under 2 years old. Treatment is supportive in a hospital. Gastric lavage or ipecac induced vomiting may help if done in time, and if the patient is adequately alert. Attention should be especially directed at maintaining adequate urinary output. Naloxone in one case has been reported to reverse sedation, as well as anticonvulsant effects of Depakote.

TEGRETAL OVERDOSE

Lower overdoses can cause AV block such that cardiac monitoring is necessary. Higher overdoses depress breathing, and can cause stupor, coma and fatality. Treatment includes gastric lavage with multiple dose activated charcoal suspension, repeatedly (even after 4 hours). Due to tegretal's enterohepatic circulation, laxatives, charcoal or resin hemoperfusion may be useful. Dialysis removes about half of Tegretal's toxic metabolite and is for severe poisoning with kidney failure or small children. Breathing and blood pressure need monitoring and possibly assisted.

KLONOPIN OVERDOSE
See Benzodiazepines

ANTIPSYCHOTIC OVERDOSE

These are 10% as dangerous as tricyclic antidepressants, yet can still cause serious problems such as low blood pressure, urinary retention, cardiac irregularity, coma, seizures, and neuroleptic malignant syndrome.
LABS: Obtain ECG, vital signs, temperature, and cardiac monitoring.
TREATMENT
Hospitalize if necessary, and watch for dystonic muscle cramp reactions. Ipecac often does not work with antipsychotics, and is not recommended. If the patient is sluggish or unconscious, gastric lavage should be started after cuffed endotracheal intubation has been done. Lavage is best if done within 4 hours of an overdose, but can help up to 36 hours after the overdose. Activated charcoal may be added (by mouth or lavage tube): Charcoal prevents further absorption.
SYMPTOMS
Low blood pressure may start in 2-3 days and progress into shock, **cardiac conduction abnormalities** (QRS, QT prolongation, ventricular arrhythmia) and heart attack. The primary treatment is fluids, secondary are pressor agents such as norepinephrine, metaraminol or phenylephrine, but not epinephrine. If low blood pressure and cardiac irregularity are with a widened QRS on ECG, intravenous sodium bicarbonate can be used as is done for tricyclic antidepressant overdose. **Obtundation** and coma can occur for 48 hours. Hemodialysis is essentially useless because of low medication concentrations. **Urinary retention** should be assumed if recent voiding has not occurred, and treated by catheterization.
Seizures occur especially in children, and should be treated with diazepam (Valium) 5-10mg intravenously. For **muscle cramps** (dystonia) give diphenhydramine (Benadryl) 0.5-1mg/kg IV or benztropine (Cogentin) 1-2mg IM. Oral doses should be continued for 24-48 hours.
Hyperthermia (severe fever) can cause brain, multi-organ, and kidney damage at 104-105.8°F or above 40-41°C. After clothes are removed, the patient can be sprayed with water, and fanned. Bromocriptine or Dantrolene can help **neuroleptic malignant syndrome** (See page 146).

COCAINE OR AMPHETAMINE OVERDOSE

Most of these are done with illegally obtained "street drugs" such as cocaine ("crack" or "freebase"), or methamphetamine ("ice"). They are often smoked, snorted, or injected. Agitation, depression, dilated pupils, hallucinations, confusion, violence and panic can occur. Seizures are the most frequent complication. Severe hypertension can cause hemorrhage (bleeding stroke) in the brain, aortic dissection and heart attack. Cardiac irregularity, loss of blood pressure, palpitations, chest pain and shock can occur. Nausea, vomiting and diarrhea may accompany abdominal cramping. Fever, seizures and coma usually precede death but sudden cardiac arrest can also occur. Many cocaine abusers get acute myocardial infarction. Dexedrine causes fatality in 50% of rats given 97mg/kg body weight.

TREATMENT

Maintain airway -**Seizures** can be treated with: diazepam (Valium) 5-10mg IV over 2-3 minutes or lorazepam (Ativan) 2-3mg IV. If seizures continue: **phenobarbital** 15-20mg/kg IV and/or **phenytoin**15mg/kg IV is given over 30 or more minutes **Hyperthermia** (fever) can be reduced by external cooling (remove clothes, spray with water, fanning). Ice water lavage and ice water enemas can be done. Agitation or **psychosis** can be treated with: **Haldol** 5mg IM (with cogentin 1mg), repeat every 2 hours, up to 20mg Haldol on first day or **Thorazine** (sedating) 25-50mg IM every 2 hours as needed or **Diazepam** 5-10mg IV (may repeat to 20 ml total). **Hypertension** is usually controlled by one of the above sedating treatments, otherwise: **Phentolamine** 1-5mg IV can be injected, or **Nifedipine** 10-20mg orally can help. **Labetalol** 10-20mg IV can be used instead. **Esmolol** 25-100 ug/kg/minute IV can be added for rapid heart rate and irregularity. Other measures: Monitoring vital signs, urine drug screen collection, and getting an ECG. **Gastric lavage** can be done, with **activated charcoal**, or the charcoal can be given alone. Do not induce vomiting because of seizure risk. The urine should be kept at a normal Ph for severe intoxication since myoglobin (due to amphetamine rhabdomyolysis) is excreted better in alkaline urine, while amphetamine is better excreted in acidic urine. Hemodialysis, peritoneal dialysis and hemoperfusion are not effective in cocaine intoxication.

BENZODIAZEPINE OVERDOSE

This causes sleepiness, staggering, confusion, slurring and coma. Reflexes are decreased. Combined with alcohol, or other depressants, the overdose is more likely to be fatal. **Vital signs** (breathing, pulse, blood pressure) should be monitored. Empty the stomach by inducing vomiting (ipecac) if alertness is adequate. Gastric lavage and activated charcoal can be administered. The **airway** and ventilation should be maintained. **Intravenous fluids** should be given. Dialysis does not help. Low **blood pressure** can be treated with: Levophed (Norepinephrine 4ml (4mg) in 1 liter of 5% dextrose solution OR Aramine - (Metaraminol 2 to 10mg IM or subcutaneously or by IV infusion 15 to 100mg in 500ml NaCl injection or 5% dextrose injection OR 0.5-5mg IV followed by above infusion). Cardiac arrest and death are rare but can occur. Flumazenil ("**Romazicon**") is not recommended as an antidote for benzodiazepine intoxication. It works well to reverse benzodiazepine anesthesia or "conscious sedation" where a therapeutic dose of benzodiazepine has been given under controlled circumstances. According to clinicians, in the overdose situation, flumazenil is not as easy to use or as effective as has been claimed by the manufacturer. Flumazenil by itself can cause seizures when given for a benzodiazepine overdose. Flumazenil often does not work at all, or for only a few minutes. If the patient is a chronic user of benzodiazepines, giving flumazenil will cause the patient to develop an acute benzodiazepine withdrawal reaction characterized by seizures. The treatment for this reaction is administration of benzodiazepines, which the patient is already overdosed on, which poses a very serious therapeutic dilemma: Phenytoin will not stop the seizures, and any GABA inhibiting drug like benzodiazepines or barbiturates are contraindicated.

THYROID AUGMENTATION MEDICINES OVERDOSE

CYTOMEL, TRIOSTAT (IV), LEVOTHROID, LEVOXYL, SYNTHROID, ARMOUR, S-P-T, THYRAR, THYROLAR

The person may feel nervous, agitated, irritable, hyperactive, fatigued, hot, sweaty, insomnic, disorganized, or disoriented. Tremor, diarrhea, vomiting, high fever, dehydration, muscle cramping, palpitations, and angina can occur. The eyes may appear to be staring. Cardiac (atrial) irregularity or rarely heart failure happen. Psychosis, confusion, seizures and coma can also occur.

Thyroid medications containing T3 are three to five times more potent than those containing T4. Symptoms of thyroid intoxication from T3 can occur within 24 hours, but symptoms from ingestion or overdose or T4 can be delayed for as long as 11 days, during which period the patient's thyroid function tests should be monitored.

Treatment

Thyroid dosage should be reduced or temporarily discontinued. After suppression, normal function by the thyroid may take 6-8 weeks.
Vomiting can be induced.
Propranolol (inderal) 20-40mg, 4 times per day or 1-3mg IV over a 10 minute period.
Benzodiazepines can calm anxiety (Xanax). Cholestyramine interferes with thyroxine absorption.
Glucocorticoids can inhibit conversion of T4 to T3. Digitalis is indicated if congestive heart failure develops.
Control of fever, hypoglycemia, and fluid loss. Oxygen and ventilation may be given.
For seizures, see page 155.

ESTROGEN OVERDOSE

No serious effects (other than nausea and vomiting) occur.

PREGNANCY AND NURSING

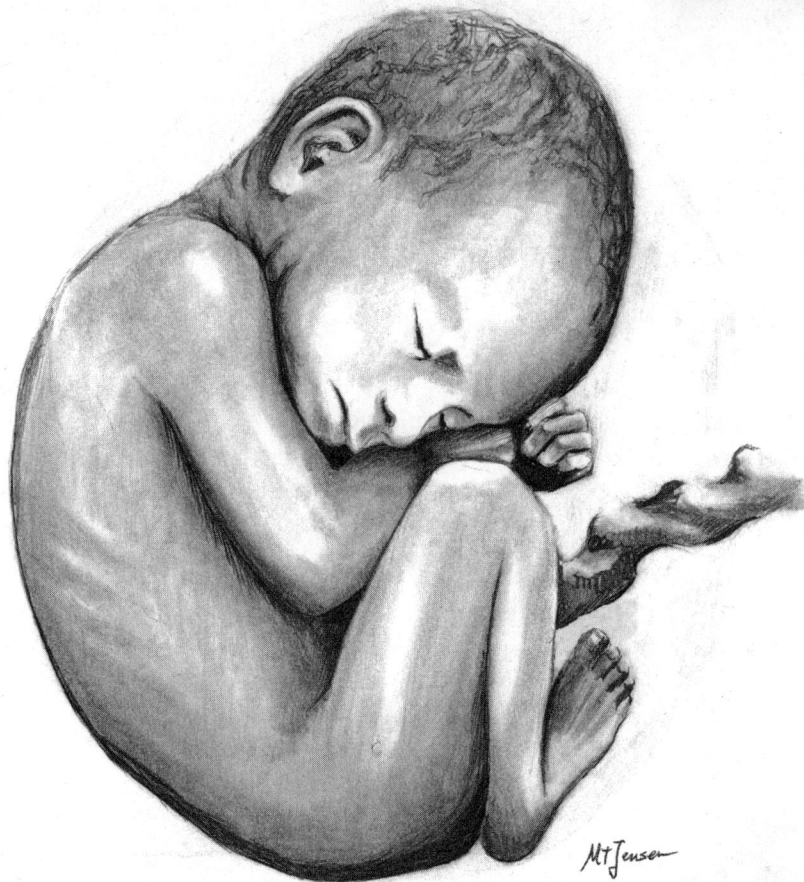

PREGNANCY AND NURSING

Unless they are absolutely needed, it is recommended all psychotropic medicines be avoided <u>during</u> pregnancy, especially the first trimester and prior to delivery. The same is recommended for nursing. If a patient discovers she is pregnant while taking a medication, she should stop it immediately. Environmental pollution worldwide may be threatening wildlife populations and perhaps humans. Adding medications during pregnancy to this already existing genetic burden should be avoided. Here is some information on the subject:

[A] Controlled studies show no risk.
[B] No evidence of risk to humans.
[C] Risk cannot be ruled out (use only if clearly needed).
[D] Positive evidence of risk.
[X] Contraindicated in pregnancy.

ANTIDEPRESSANTS

Tricyclic antidepressants have much data, and for most, no major problems have been identified. Animal studies are inconclusive. Tricyclics pass into the breast milk, and have variable concentration there. They may not cause significant plasma levels or toxicity in the infant. The medications should be tapered 5-10 days before delivery to avoid infant withdrawal syndromes. If a mother wants to take antidepressant while nursing, the infant should be observed closely. According to several sources, **MAOI's** have been shown to be clearly harmful to animal fetuses. Details on the antidepressants follow alphabetically:

ADAPIN - See Sinequan.

ANAFRANIL   Clomipramine   [C]
Slight toxic effects occurred on embryos of rats given 5-10 times the maximum human dose. Tremor and seizures can occur in a newborn if the mother was taking anafranil, and didn't taper it off before delivery. The medicine does enter breast milk

ASCENDIN   Amoxapin   [C]
Death of the fetus, stillbirth and decreased birth weight were seen in animals getting 3-20 times the human dose. Decreased survival in the first 4 days in rat offspring occurred.
Nursing: Most systemic drugs enter breast milk.

DESYREL   Trazadone   [C]
In rats at 30-50 times the maximum human dose, this causes various adverse effects including the fetus absorbing into the mother. In rabbits, congenital abnormalities occurred at doses 15-50 times the maximum. On nursing, there is no data.

EFFEXOR   Venlafaxine   [C]
There are no studies involving women, but rats and rabbits given 11 and 12 times the maximum human dose revealed no malformations. However, rats had decreased pup weights, increased stillbirths, and increased pup deaths during the first 5 days of life. The safe dose concerning rat pup mortality was 1.4 times the human dose. No data is available on nursing. Most drugs are excreted in human milk.

ELAVIL   Amitriptyline   [C]
There have been a few reports of limb deformities and   developmental delays when mothers took this during pregnancy. Mice, rats and rabbits at 13 times the maximum dose had no deformities. Mice and hamsters at 33 times the maximum dose had multiple deformities. A rat study at 8 times maximum dose showed delays in bone hardening. Nursing: In one report the mother's serum Elavil level was similar to the level in her breast milk, but this was not enough to cause any serum level in the infant.

162

ENDEP - See Elavil.

LUDIOMIL Maprotiline [B]
Studies in rabbits, mice and rats at doses of 1.3, 7, and 9 times the human maximum dose revealed no evidence of harm to the animal fetuses. The medication is excreted in breast milk at a concentration that corresponds to the serum level.

LUVOX Fluvoxamine [C]
In rats and rabbits, at twice the human dose, there were no malformations. Other studies, however, suggested these doses and higher could increase pup mortality and decrease weight.

NARDIL Phenelzine -MAOI [C]
In high dose, this has adverse effects in mice. They show a significant reduction in the number of viable offspring. The growth of young dogs and rats has been slowed by this medication. Nursing is not recommended with this.

NORPRAMINE Desipramine [C]
Animal studies are inconclusive. This antidepressant, as well as Nortriptyline, have been favored.

PAMELAR Nortriptyline [D]
Animal studies are inconclusive. This antidepressant, as well as Desipramine have been favored. Yet rare limb abnormalities have developed in the children of mothers taking Nortriptyline while pregnant.

PARNATE Tranylcypromine -MAOI [C]
This has not been demonstrated to be safe to animal fetuses. It passes into breast milk. Nursing is not recommended with this.

PAXIL Paroxetine [B]
There are no studies involving women, but rats and rabbits given up to 50 and 6 times the maximum human dose revealed no harm to the fetus. This is secreted into human milk. Effects on infants are unknown.

PROZAC Fluoxetine [B]
There are no studies that have been done involving women, but rats and rabbits given 9 and 11 times the maximum human dose (80mg.) revealed no evidence of harm to the fetus. In one breast milk sample, the Prozac was 1/4 the concentration found in the mother's blood.

SERZONE Nefazodone [C]
Rats and rabbits given 5 and 6 times the maximum human dose had no malformations. Rat pups however had increased mortality and lower weight. No problems occurred at 1.3 times the human dose.

SINEQUAN Doxepin [C]
Studies in rats, rabbits, monkeys and dogs show no evidence of harm to the fetus. There has been one report of drowsiness and poor breathing in a nursing infant whose mother was taking Sinequan.

SURMONTIL Trimipramine [C]
Increased major abnormalities occur in rats and rabbits at 20 times the maximum human dose.

TOFRANIL Imipramine [D]
Rat studies at 2-1/2 times the maximum human dose indicate that litter size and birth weight are reduced while rate of stillbirths is increased. In humans, limb abnormalities rarely have developed. Mothers taking this medicine should not nurse.

VIVACTIL Protriptyline [C]
No data is available for humans. In mice, rats and rabbits, doses 10 times greater than human doses had no harmful effects on reproduction.

WELLBUTRIN   Bupropion   [B]
In rats and rabbits getting 15-45 times the human dose, there was no evidence of harm. Yet in rabbits, 2 studies showed an increase in fetal abnormalities. On nursing, there is no information, but Wellbutrin is remarkable for seizure risk in adults.

ZOLOFT   Sertraline   [B]
There are no studies involving women, but rats and rabbits given 20 and 10 times the maximum human dose showed no deformities. At doses as low as 2.5 times the maximum dose, animal fetuses had delayed formation of bone. At 5 times the maximum dose to the mother, newborn animals had decreased survival. No data is available on nursing.

MOOD STABILIZERS: PREGNANCY / NURSING

LITHIUM   [D]
This may cause fetal harm in humans if taken during pregnancy. Data suggests deformities at a rate of 12%. This includes malformations of the heart, nervous system and outer ear. Yet many healthy babies have been born from mothers who received lithium throughout the pregnancy. Lithium should, if possible, be discontinued 1-2 months prior to conception, and be avoided, especially, the first trimester of pregnancy as well as 2-3 days prior to delivery.

Newborn or nursing infants exposed to lithium can be limp, tired, and bluish in color due to lack of adequate breathing. Lithium enters the breast milk at a concentration of 10-100% of the mother's serum lithium level. Lithium treated mothers should not nurse their infants. Women receiving lithium can use birth control and plan pregnancies carefully. If pregnancy occurs, the lithium should be stopped. If lithium exposure in pregnancy occurred before the 12th week of pregnancy, cardiac ultrasound can be done at 16-20 weeks gestation to check for heart abnormalities.

Carbamazapine (Tegretal) may be sometimes used in place of lithium the first trimester. It is usually less effective. Since this is also somewhat toxic, electric shock therapy can be considered if symptoms are dangerous. If the pregnant mother chooses to go without any medicines, a neuroleptic (see that section) can be used as needed to control severe symptoms. Psychotic women risk fetal loss much more than normal women.

DEPAKOTE   Divalproex   [D]
This may cause fetal harm in humans at a rate of 4-5% if taken during the first trimester of pregnancy. Malformations can be in the nervous system, skeleton and heart. Cleft lip, bleeding defects, liver failure, and growth deficiency can also occur in the fetus.
The breast milk contains 1-10% the concentration of what is in the mother's serum.

TEGRETAL   Carbamazapine   [C]
This is almost devoid of malformation risk though anticonvulsant medications have an overall rate of 4-5% for malformations. In general, face and head defects, underdeveloped nails and growth delays can occur in fetuses. Concentration in breast milk is 25-60% that of mother's serum.

KLONOPIN   Clonazepam   [C]
In rats given about 30 times the maximum human dose, there were fewer pregnancies, and more offspring dying before weaning. Pregnant rabbits given varying doses, including some in the human range had limb defects, cleft palates and open eyelids, without regard to dose. A few rabbits were vulnerable at all doses, while others were not, at any dose.
Most closely resembles benzodiazepines.

INDERAL   Propranolol   [C]
(for lithium tremor)
This is toxic to embryos in animals, at 10 times the human dose. Caution should be exercised when nursing because this enters breast milk.

164

Some patients require this during pregnancy. If possible these medicines should be avoided during the period of highest risk (4-10 weeks after conception). The anti-psychotic should, if possible, be stopped 2 weeks prior to delivery to minimize excessive crying, and medication side effect symptoms in the new-born. Resume antipsy-chotics immediately after delivery. Antipsychotics do pass into breast milk.

Any of these choices are felt to be safest because they are potent and can be used in low doses:
    Fluphenazine   (Prolixin)
    Haloperidol   (Haldol)
    Perphenazine   (Trilafon)
    Trifluoperazine (Stelazine)

Details on the neuroleptics follow, alphabetically:

CLOZARIL   Clozapine   [B]
In rats and rabbits given 2-4 times the human dose, there have been no adverse effects or impaired fertility. This enters breast milk, so these mothers should not nurse.

HALOPERIDOL   Haldol   [C]
At 2-20 times the maximum human dose, rodents showed decreased fertility, increased absorption of fetuses into the mother, delayed deliveries, and more pup mortality. Infants of mothers taking this should not be nursed.

LOXITANE   Loxapine   [C]
Studies have shown in rats treated from mid-pregnancy on, at doses approximating a usual human level, that structural changes occurred in the kidneys of offspring. This was below the maximum recommended human dose. Mothers taking this medicine should avoid nursing if possible.

MELLARIL   Thioridazine   [C]
Studies in animals have shown no malformation effect.

MOBAN   Molindone   [C]
In animal studies, no malformations have been seen. Rats and rabbits had no effects, but mice showed slight absorption of fetuses into the mothers. No data is available on nursing.

NAVANE   Thiothixene   [C]
In animals, there is a decrease in fertility and litter size. Rats and rabbits showed increased absorption of fetuses into the mother. No malformations have been seen in these animals, or in monkeys given about 4 times the maximum human dose.

ORAP   Pimozide   [C]
In rabbits given 8 times the maximum human dose, harm to embryos occurred. Offspring had more frequent death, and lower weights.

PROLIXIN   Fluphenazine   [C]
"Safety has not yet been established": No negative studies were located by me.

RISPERDAL   Risperidone   [C]
In rats and rabbits, at 6 times the human dose, there was no increase in malformations. In rats, at 0.1 to 3 times the human dose, there were increased pup deaths and stillbirths. There is one report of an infant being born missing a part of the brain ("corpus callosum"), whose mother took this medicine while pregnant. A mother taking this should not nurse.

SERENTIL   Mesoridazine   [C]
"Safety has not yet been established": No negative studies were located by me.

STELAZINE   Trifluoperazine   [C]

There are some reports of newborns having medication side effects ("EPS") and increased or decreased reflexes. There is also a longer period of yellowish discoloration in the newborn. Rat offspring show increased malformations, reduced weight and reduced liter size when rat mothers are given 600 times the human dose. At 300 times the human dose, this was not seen. No adverse effects to offspring were seen in rabbits given 700 times the human dose, nor in monkeys receiving 25 times the human dose. This medicine is excreted in breast milk.

TARACTIN   Chloprothixene   [C]

Rats receiving about the equivalent of a full human dose had an increased rate of stillbirths, and absorption of embryos into the mother. Rabbits had no problems at 1 and 2 times the maximum human dose.

THORAZINE   Chlorpromazine   [C]

There are some reports of newborns having medication side effects ("EPS"), and increased or decreased reflexes. There is also a longer period of yellowish discoloration in the newborn. In rodents there is toxicity to the embryo, and increased newborn deaths. Offspring have diminished performance and possibly permanent brain injury. This medicine is excreted in breast milk.

TRILAFON   Perphenazine   [C]

"Safety has not yet been established": No negative studies were located by me.

SIDE EFFECT MEDICINES FOR ANTIPSYCHOTICS, LITHIUM

AKINETON   Biperiden   [C]

Effects are unknown concerning fetal risk and nursing.

ARTANE   Trihexyphenidyl   [C]

There is no apparent fetal risk if a mother takes this during pregnancy.

BENADRYL   Diphenhydramine   [B]

Studies with rats and rabbits at 5 times the human dose revealed no harm to fetuses. Human studies have not been done.

COGENTIN   Benztropine   [C]

There is no apparent fetal risk if a mother takes this during pregnancy.

DANTRIUM   Dantrolene   [C]

Safety during pregnancy has not been established. This should not be used in nursing mothers.

INDERAL   Propranolol   [C]

This is toxic to embryos in animals, at 10 times the human dose. Caution should be exercised when nursing because this enters breast milk.

KEMADRIN   Procyclidine   [C]

Safety has not been established for pregnancy or nursing.

PARLODEL   Bromocriptine   [C]

This has a 3.3% rate of malformations (limbs, hip, etc.) and an 11% incidence of spontaneous abortions. Yet these are essentially the same rates that occur in the general population.

SYMMETREL   Amantadine   [C]

In rats this harms embryos and causes malformations at 12 times the human dose. Rabbits getting 25 times the human dose had no toxic effects. The medicine enters breast milk and the mother.

STIMULANTS: PREGNANCY / NURSING

RITALIN   Methylphenidate   [C]
Animal studies have not been conducted. This should not taken by pregnant women until more is known.

DEXEDRINE / DEXTROSTAT   Dextroamphetamine   [C]
In mice, at 41 times the maximum human dose, this is toxic to embryos and can cause malformations. Rabbits given 7 times the human dose, and rabbits given 12.5 times the maximum dose had no toxic effects on the embryo.

Infants born to mothers addicted to amphetamines have low birth weight and more premature delivery. After being born, they can show withdrawal distress, agitation and tiredness. Stimulants enter breast milk, so mothers taking this should not nurse.

CATAPRES   Clonidine   [C]
Rabbits given 3 times the maximum human dose had no evidence of fetal harm. Rats, however, showed increased reabsorptions of the fetuses. The medicine enters breast milk.

CYLERT   Pemoline   [B]
No malformations have been seen in rats and rabbits getting doses approximately 4 and 9 times the human dose. Rats however showed more stillbirths. Offspring survival was reduced at the same dose ranges.

IONAMIN   Phentermine resin   [C]
Safe use has not been established.

TENUATE   Diethylpropion   [B]
Rats receiving 9 times the human dose had no evidence of fetal harm. Since this medicine enters breast milk, caution should be used concerning nursing.

DESOXYN   Methamphetamine   [C]
This is abused "on the streets", and probably is 25 times more powerful than the other stimulants (power ratio of epinephrine to norepinephrine). In mammals given high doses, this kills embryos and causes malformations. Infants have low birth weight and premature birth. After being born, they also have withdrawal distress, agitation and tiredness.

ANXIETY REDUCERS AND SLEEPERS (BENZODIAZEPINES):

Most of these are for anxiety, several are sleep medications. These should be **stopped if pregnancy** is discovered, and preferably 1-2 months before attempting to conceive. Benzodiazepines generally produce high rates of malformation, especially during the first trimester. Trying protocols 1-3, prior to pregnancy, can frequently identify the chemical imbalance, such that safer medications can be used. If a benzodiazepine must be given, it should not be given until after the tenth week of pregnancy to avoid mouth deformities. These medications in the mother also suppress a baby's breathing at **birth**. The baby can appear limp, cool, and feed poorly. This can be followed in the newborn by a **drug withdrawal syndrome** of irritability, diarrhea, vomiting and high pitched crying. Thus if a benzodiazepine was used in the second and third trimesters, it should be tapered and stopped at least several weeks before delivery.

If **breast feeding** occurs from a benzodiazepine medicated mother, the infant becomes sluggish and looses weight. A nursing mother using phenobarbital instead, results in an alert, unaffected infant. Yet phenobarbital during pregnancy can cause fetal damage and abnormalities.

167

ANXIETY MEDICINES

ATIVAN   Lorazapam   [D]
Occasional serious malformations were seen in offspring of drug treated rabbits **unrelated to dosage** (smaller limbs, rotated limbs, unshaped skull, small eyes, etc.). At high doses there was increased rabbit fetal loss.

BUSPAR   Buspirone   [B]
This is not a benzodiazepine. No fetal damage was seen in rats and rabbits given 30 times the maximum human dose. Fertility also was normal. Nursing while taking Buspar should be avoided since effects are unknown

CENTRAX   Prazepam   [C]
This has not been studied adequately. It may be similar to other benzodiazepines concerning a risk of infant malformations if taken by the mother during the first trimester.

KLONOPIN   Clonazepam   [C]
In rats given about 30 times the maximum human dose, there were fewer pregnancies, and more offspring dying before weaning. Pregnant rabbits given varying doses, including some in the human range had limb defects, cleft palates and open eyelids, without regard to dose. A few rabbits were vulnerable at all doses, while others were not, at any dose.

LIBRIUM   Chlordiazepoxide   [D]
One study found an 11% incidence of congenital abnormalities. A rat study showed major skeletal defects can occur in offspring if the mother receives this medication during pregnancy.

SERAX   Oxazepam   [C]
This has not been studied adequately. It may be similar to other benzodiazepines concerning a risk of infant malformations if taken by the mother during the first trimester. Breeding medicated rats through two liters resulted in no fetal malformations.

TRANXENE   Chlorazepate   [C]
This has not been studied adequately. It may be similar to other benzodiazepines concerning a risk of infant malformations if taken by the mother during the first trimester. Yet rats and rabbits given about 100 and 10 times the maximum human dose produced no abnormalities in the fetuses. This medicine also is excreted in breast milk.

VALIUM   Diazepam   [D]
Rats showed decreased surviving offspring and fewer pregnancies. Some studies showed new-born rats had skeletal and other defects. One human study found that of children with cleft palate, 6% of the mothers had used this medicine the first trimester. Another rat study using Valium at about 100 times the human dose resulted in no malformations. Valium can cause malformations if given the first trimester.

XANAX   Alprazolam   [D]
Because this is a benzodiazepine, it is capable of causing a risk of malformations if the mother takes it during the first trimester. It may cause fetal harm including clubfoot, turned ankle, hernia, tongue-tie, and stomach closure ("pyloric stenosis").

SLEEPER MEDICINES

Most of these are benzodiazepines with an even higher rate of damage to fetuses.

AMBIEN   Zolpidem   [B]
In rats and rabbits, no toxic effects were seen at 5 and 7 times the maximum human dose. In rats at doses 25 and 125 times, and in rabbits at 20 times the maximum human dose, there were delays in bone hardening. Using this during nursing is not recommended.

DALMANE   Flurazepam   [X]
Benzodiazepines may cause fetal damage when given during pregnancy. A newborn was inactive and limp four days following birth because the mother took this nightly before delivery.

DORAL   Quazepam   [X]
Benzodiazepines may cause fetal damage when given during pregnancy.

HALCION   Triazolam   [X]
A single dose to the mother in the first trimester can cause multiple abnormalities. This is secreted in breast milk, so nursing mothers should not receive this.

PROZOM   Estazolam   [X]
Benzodiazepines may cause fetal damage when given during pregnancy.

RESTORIL   Temazepam   [X]
Benzodiazepines may cause fetal damage when given during pregnancy. Rat and rabbit studies using about 100 times the maximum human dose showed skeletal malformations.

THYROID AUGMENTATION MEDICINES [A]

CYTOMEL, TRIOSTAT (IV), LEVOTHROID, LEVOXYL, SYNTHROID, ARMOUR, S-P-T, THYRAR, THYROLAR

These hormones do not easily cross the placental barrier. No adverse effect has been found on fetuses when mothers take thyroid during pregnancy.

Small amounts of thyroid hormone are excreted in breast milk, and no reactions have been noted in nursing babies. Thyroid replacement treatment is needed to maintain breast feeding in hypothyroid mothers.

ESTROGEN [X]

Estrogen should not be used during pregnancy. Male offspring can have reproductive tract abnormalities. Female offspring are at increased risk for cancer later in life.

CHAPTER
12

GLOSSARY for Patients

GLOSSARY FOR PATIENTS

ADD, ADHD: Attention deficit disorder, attention deficit hyperactivity disorder, used interchangeably with DA/NE failure. See page 19 for symptoms

Adrenal Glands: These are on top of each kidney in the back of the abdomen. The surface makes steroids, and the interior makes "catacholamines" which are epinephrine and norepinephrine, the fight or flight hormones. These last 5-10 times as long as the norepinephrine secreted by the brain, and epinephrine increases metabolism 5-10 times more strongly than the NE.

Adrenergic: Substances which are adrenaline-like: Epinephrine, Norepinephrine, or medicines which stimulate the receptors for these substances causing energization in normal people, or calming in A.D.D. patients, who may have a failure in this system. Patients with NE instability, electrical instability or dopamine elevation may get worse with adrenergic substances.

Agoraphobia: Fear of situations where escape is difficult, for example anywhere outside of home, crowds, freeways, standing in a line etc. Due to the same variety of chemistries that cause anxiety (see page 53).

Akathisia: Possible antipsychotic medication side effects of restlessness, anxiety and inability to sit still.

Amphetamine: As a drug, this has been abused in powerful concentrated forms. As a medication this has worked to possibly replace a deficiency of a similar substance (DA/NE) that is missing or failing in the brain of some patients. In this situation it can fix hyperactivity, anxiety, depression or poor concentration, without causing tolerance or addiction.

Antagonist: A medicine that nullifies the action of another medicine. Receptor binding occurs, but there is no reaction. Thus the site is occupied and blocked from functioning.

Anticholinergic: Dryness of mouth, blurring and constipation side effects of some antidepressants, antipsychotics and side effect medicines.

Anticonvulsants: Medicines that stabilize seizures in epileptics, and unstable electricity in patients with mood problems.

Anxietolytics: Medicines that decrease anxiety and tension.

Benzodiazepines: These medicines (such as Valium and Xanax - "Benzos") can be addictive, especially at higher doses, but help to decrease anxiety. Many other medicines can neutralize anxiety (see page 53).

Beta (adrenergic) blocker: These medicines block epinephrine and norepinephrine effects. B_1 receptors help heart rate, contractility and oxygen flow to the lungs. Beta receptors become excessive in panic disorder.

Bipolar: Synonymous with manic depression. See page 18.
Many people have this chemistry without the classic symptoms.

BUN: The "blood urea nitrogen" increases if the kidneys are failing, or the urinary tract is obstructed. Urea is a waste product of protein metabolism.

CBC: The "complete blood count" includes the hemoglobin and hematocrit which detects anemia, and the white blood cell count which detects infection, certain cancers, and immune functioning.

Cognitive Therapy: A directive type of therapy that is based on the belief that emotional problems are mainly caused by distorted attitudes that can be corrected.

Creatinine: A metabolic waste product excreted in the urine that is useful in measuring kidney function.

172

Creatinine Phosphokinase (CPK): An enzyme found in muscles, the brain and the heart. This becomes elevated in neuroleptic malignant syndrome. See page146.

DA/NE Failure: Dopamine/Norepinephrine failure is a chemical description I made to describe attention deficit disorder (see page 19). This can occur without A.D.D. symptoms, and can cause depression or panic.

Destabilizers: Substances which cause worsening of various chemical imbalances, and thus make the person who took the substance feel worse.

Detoxification: Medical treatment to help an addict withdraw from a drug or alcohol habit.

Dopamine: A chemical with many different functions depending on where in the body it occurs. In one area of the brain, elevation causes hallucinations.

DSM-4: The Diagnostic and Statistical Manual for Mental Disorders
(4th edition) is a compilation by a task force of 25 physicians, describing approximately 370 psychiatric categories.

Electricity Smoothing: A term I made to describe the action of anticonvulsant seizure medicines that stabilize electrical instability, and thus correct mood instability, and other symptoms.

Fluid Aggressive Trial & Error: A treatment approach which is flexible and active. It is a recognition by me that I cannot recognize chemical imbalance types until they are medically proven by good results. See the graphs in chapter IV.

FTI: The "Free Thyroxin Index" measures thyroid functioning and correlates with the Free T_4. It is the product of "total T_4 and T_3RU," and corrects for TBG (thyroid binding globulin) variation. TBG can be high with pregnancy, oral contraceptives, liver disease, phenothiazines, or genetically.

GABA: Gamma-aminobutyric acid is a brain chemical which inhibits other neurotransmitters. It generally relaxes anxiety.

Half Life: How long a medication takes to be half eliminated from the body.

Hemoperfusion: Similar to dialysis to remove lethal levels of a drug overdose from the blood. Special chemical columns are used.

Hypothyroidism: Low thyroid functioning which causes a low metabolic rate. See page 47 for symptoms.

Interstitial Cystitis: An inflammatory lesion of the bladder wall, usually in women. Urination is frequent, and pain occurs with a full bladder, and at the end of urination.

Labile: Mood overactivity and instability.

Leukocytosis: Increased white blood cells resulting from infection, fever, inflammation or hemorrhage (severe bleeding).

MAOI: Monoamine oxidase inhibitors are antidepressants that are strong, but more hazardous.

NE: See Norepinephrine

Neuroleptic Malignant Syndrome: A toxic and dangerous reaction that can occur especially when antipsychotic dosage is raised too fast. See page 146.

Neuroleptics: Antipsychotic medication, blocks dopamine.

Neuronal: Pertaining to nerves (neurons).

Neurotransmitter System: Any one of a group of substances released or sensed by nerves in the brain. These effect mood and behavior. See page 15.

Norepinephrine: This is a major neurotransmitter that can be unstable, low, or failing, resulting in a wide variety of symptoms. High NE causes mania, low NE causes depression or panic. Failed DA/NE causes attention deficit disorder.

Norepinephrine receptors: All brain transmitter chemicals are released by a given nerve. Another nerve, the "receptor" then reacts to that brain transmitter chemical. In some panic disorders, there is an excess of NE receptors causing anxiety.

Obtundation: Almost unconscious.

Organicity: This term is used loosely here to denote emotions which are due to lesions or medical illness.

Perfectionistic: A disposition of unusual meticulousness and organization.

Pharmacologic: Relating to medications.

PR Interval: A portion of the electrocardiogram which reflects conduction from the atrium to the ventricle of the heart. With tricyclic antidepressants, this is prolonged.

Psychosis: Severe impairment of senses resulting in confusion, hallucinations, paranoia, delusions, incoherence and agitation. Usually is due to elevated dopamine.

Psychotropics: Medications which can modify mental activity, emotions, or feelings.

QT/QRS Widening: On an electrocardiogram, this indicates that tricyclic antidepressant toxicity is occurring. See page 156, 175.

Reactivity: A term I use to describe a chemical imbalance whose exact identity is unknown, but which reacts adversely to antidepressants given to the patient. This usually signifies undelying circuits from protocol 2-4 are present. The question is whether a protocol 1 medicine exists that won't aggrevate the circuit.

Reticulocyte Count: A reticulocyte is a young red blood cell. Counting these clarifies if the bone marrow is healthy and not being injured.

Schizophrenia: Psychotic disorders with bizarre speech, hallucinations, delusions, flattened or inappropriate moods, or paranoia. See page 19.

Serotonin: This is a major neurotransmitter that when low can cause a variety of mental symptoms, but especially perfectionism, pain, and tension.

SMA 25: "Sequential Multiple Analyzer" is a trademark for a blood test which checks 25 substances in the blood to screen for illness in various systems of the body.

SNRI: Selective serotonin and norepinephrine reuptake inhibitor is an antidepressant that has a strong and specific enhancement towards serotonin and norepinephrine.

Somnolence: Sleepiness, sedation.

Spansule: A long acting form of a medicine.

SSRI: A Selective Serotonin Reuptake Inhibitor has a strong and specific action to enhance serotonin.

ST Depression: On the electrocardiogram, this is useful to analyze toxicity of tricyclic antidepressants.
T-Wave: See diagram below (electrocardiogram).

T4: Thyroxine is the major hormone made by the thyroid gland. It has 4 iodines per molecule, and is converted in the bodies tissues to a more active, potent form called "T_3."

Tardive Dyskinesia: Abnormal, sometimes irreversible movements (usually chewing) that can occur from usually high dose, prolonged antipsychotic treatment. See page 145.

TCA: Tricyclic antidepressants—can be very effective in correcting serotonin and/or NE, but are more dangerous in overdosage.

Titrate: Careful adjustment of medication to relieve symptoms.

Tourettes: A neurologic genetic disorder with motor tics (squinting, grimacing, tongue protrusion) and vocal tics (throat clearing, clicks, swearing) worsened by stress.

TSH: Thyroid stimulating hormone is high or low with thyroid failure or excess.

UA: Urinalysis

VDRL: Test for syphilis. See page 110.

WBC: The white blood cell count is useful in assessing if infection, allergy or immune failure are occurring.

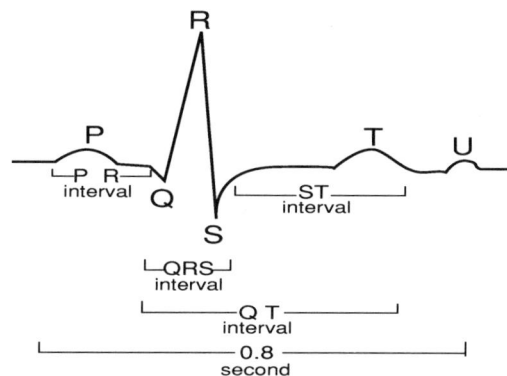

Normal Electrocardiogram of Heart

MEDICINE INDEX

MEDICINES / SUBSTANCES	ACTIONS (Follow Brand Names)
Adapin / doxepin	Sedating antidepressant, half out in 17 hours.
Akineton / biperiden	Stops antipsychotic side effects. See page 72.
Alcohol / Ethanol	Affects GABA and is used socially. Peaks in 30 to 90 minutes. Half life is 14 minutes, but a maximum of 1oz. (30ml) is cleared every 3 hours. Can be addictive.
Alprazolam / **Xanax**	
Amantadine / **Symmetrel**	
Ambien / zolpidem	Very gentle GABA sleeper. Peaks in 1.5 hours, half gone in about 3 hours.
Amitriptyline / **Elavil**, **Endep**	
Amoxapine / **Ascendin**	
Amphetamine	A class of medication that in low dosage, can be safe to stimulate or replace DA / NE for attention deficit disorder chemistry. However, when abused (pills, snorting, smoking, injecting), this is addictive, especially at higher dose ranges. Tolerance often develops to the anorexic effects of diet pills. Yet A.D.D. and some medically ill patients do not get tolerant or addicted to this when prescribed correctly. Amphetamine for fatigue may be inappropriate, except with narcolepsy.
Anafranil / clomipramine	Antidepressant with some serotonin and NE effects. Peaks in 4 hours, but is still half in system at 96 hours. In my practice it has frequent adverse side effects. Yet it can decrease sex drive in offenders.
Antabuse / disulfiram	Causes adverse reaction with alcohol and is used to help alcoholics not drink for up to 14 days after a dose.
Armour	Thyroid augmentation medicine with mixture of T_4 and T_3 (4:1).
Artane / trihexyphenidyl	Stops antipsychotic side effects, see page 72.
Ascendin / amoxapin	A NE activating antidepressant with dopamine reducing antipsychotic action. Peaks in 1.5 hours, half gone in 8 hours.
Atenolol / **Tenormin**	
Ativan / lorazepam	Calms anxiety by GABA enhancement (benzodiazepine). Peaks in 2 hours, half gone in 14 hours.
Baclofen / **Lioresal**	
Benadryl / diphenhydramine	Stops antipsychotic side effects, and is an antihistamine. Peaks in 1 hour, half gone in 8 hours. See Page 72.

Bentyl / dicyclomine	Relieves bowel cramping during opiate withdrawal.
Benzodiazepine	A class of medication that enhances GABA and calms anxiety, but at higher doses especially, can be addictive and effect coordination.
Benztropine / **Cogentin**	
Bethanechol / **Urecholine**	
Biperiden / **Akineton**	
Bromocriptine / **Parlodel**	
Bupropion / **Wellbutrin**	
Buspar / buspirone	Effects serotonin and dopamine, sometimes helps anxiety. Peaks in 40-90 minutes, half gone in 2.5 hours.
Buspirone / **Buspar**	
Caffeine (coffee)	This may increase NE. Caffeine is half gone in about 5 hours. See page 119.
Carbamazepine / **Tegretal**	
Catapres / clonidine	Good for opiate withdrawal to decrease adrenaline like symptoms. May help some hyperactive children's misbehavior. It is a blood pressure pill, peaks in 4 hours, half gone in 14 hours.
Chloral Hydrate	Barbiturate like substance sometimes used as a sleeper during heroin detoxification. Half gone in 8 hours.
Chlordiazepoxide / **Librium**	
Chlorpromazine / **Thorazine**	
Chlorprothixene / **Taractin**	
Choline	May help tardive dyskinesia
Clomipramine / **Anafranil**	
Clonazepam / **Klonopin**	
Clonidine / **Catapres**	
Clorazepate / **Tranxene**	
Clozapine / **Clozaril**	
Clozaril / clozapine	An effective antipsychotic for when all others have failed. It can be used safely if weekly blood test monitoring is done.
Cocaine	("crack" is similar) Causes temporary dopamine /norepinephrine increase followed by possible brain injury and destabilization. Highly addictive. Half gone in 50 minutes.

Cogentin / benztropine	Stops antipsychotic side effects, see page 72.
Cylert / pemoline	This is an altered amphetamine that is practically not abusable. Peaks in 3 hours, half gone in 12 hours.
Cytomel / liothyronine	This thyroid augmentation (T_3) is sometimes too potent and activating or destabilizing. Half gone in 2.5 days.
Dalmane / flurazepam	Benzodiazepine GABA sleeper, strong and long acting. Peaks in 30-60 minutes, but is only half gone in 74 hours.
Dantrium / dantroline	For neuroleptic malignant syndrome.
Dantroline / **Dantrium**	
Depakote / divalproex	Stabilizes unstable electricity and moods. Peaks in 3- 4 hours, half gone in 11 hours.
Desipramine / **Norpramine**	
Desoxyn / methamphetamine	Resembles epinephrine which is 5-10 times more powerful then NE, and so is abused more. Amphetamine.
Desyrel / trazadone	A serotonin antidepressant that is gentle and short acting. Peaks in 1.5 hours, half gone in 6 hours. It is often a useful non-addictive sleep medicine for females, but males can get erections that may require surgery (page 136).
Dexedrine / dextroamphetamine	See amphetamine. Half gone in 10 hours.
Dextrostat / dextroamphetamine	See amphetamine. Half gone in 10 hours.
Diazepam / **Valium**	
Dicyclomine / **Bentyl**	
Diethylpropion / **Tenuate**	
Dilantin / phenytoin	A seizure medicine that stabilizes electricity. It may raise serotonin, NE, dopamine, and at higher levels GABA. Peaks in 4-12 hours, half gone in 22 hours.
Disulfiram / **Antabuse**	
Divalproex / **Depakote**	
Dopa	An amino acid that is converted to dopamine, then norepin-ephrine, then epinephrine.
Doral / quazepam	Benzodiazepine GABA sleeper, peaks in 2 hours, half gone in 56 hours.
Doxepin / **Sinequan** / **Adapin**	
Effexor / venlafaxine	A potent serotonin-norepinephrine antidepressant (SNRI) - looks similar to prozac, but is shorter acting. It is half gone in 8 hours and is activating.

Elavil / amitriptyline	A sedating antidepressant. Peaks in 7 hours, half gone in 22 hours.
Eskalith / lithium	Brand name lithium, this stabilizes mood probably by stabilizing NE. Peaks in 1 / 2 - 2 hours and is half gone in 22 hours. Eskalith CR" peaks in 4-6 hours.
Estazolam / **Prosom**	
Ethanol / alcohol	
Etraphon / perphenazine-amitriptyline	Serotonin correcting antidepressant with antipsychotic component.
Fluoxetine / **Prozac**	
Fluphenazine / **Prolixin**	
Flurazepam / **Dalmane**	
Fluvoxamine / **Luvox**	
Habitrol	Each skin patch delivers nicotine for 24 hours to help smokers stop their habit. Less morning craving.
Halcion / triazolam	A short acting effective GABA sleep medicine (benzodiazepine). Peaks in 2 hours, half gone in 3.5 hours.
Haldol / haloperidol	Excellent antipsychotic for severe psychosis, but usually is given with cogentin to prevent muscle cramps. Half gone in 18 hours.
Haloperidol / **Haldol**	
Heroin	Opiate, highly addictive, half gone in 30 minutes.
Hydroxyzine / **Vistaril**	
Imipramine / **Tofranil**	
Inderal / propranolol	Beta $_{1,2}$ blocker that decreases palpitations, tremor, migraines and hypertension. Peaks in 1-1.5 hours, half gone in 4 hours.
Ionamin / phentermine resin	A diet pill that is a mild amphetamine that resembles dexadrine structurally and can be useful for ADHD chemistry. A once daily dosage is convenient. Lasts 10-14 hours.
Kemadrin / procyclidine	Side effect medicine for antipsychotics (page 72).
Klonopin / clonazepam	A benzodiazepine that resembles ativan structurally. For seizures, this may work only temporarily. For tension can be effective in low dosage, but sometimes is sedating. Peaks in 1-4 hours, half gone in 23 hours.
Levodopa	Converted into dopamine after transport into brain; helps Parkinsonian symptoms, and tardive dyskinesia (page 145).

Levothyroxine / **Levoxin, Synthroid, Levothroid**

Levoxyl / levothyroxine	Thyroid medicine (T_4), half gone in 6 days.
Librium / chlordiazepoxide	GABA enhancement, benzodiazepine that feels dull. Peaks in 0.5 - 4 hours, half gone in 24-48 hours.
Lioresal / baclofen	Relaxes muscle spasm rigidity, and may help tardive dyskinesia.
Liothyronine / **Cytomel**	
Lithium	Norepinephrine stabilizer. Peaks in 0.5 - 2 hours, half gone in 22 hours.
Lithobid	Brand name Lithium. Peaks in 4-6 hours and is half gone in 22 hours.
Lithonate / lithium	See above.
Lithotabs / lithium	See above.
Lorazepam / **Ativan**	
Loxapine / **Loxitane**	
Loxitane / loxapine	Antipsychotic
Luvox / fluvoxamine	A potent serotonin antidepressant (SSRI) that peaks in 3-8 hours, and is half gone in 16 hours.
LSD	Drastically reduces discharges by a serotonin area of the brain causing hallucinations and tolerance.
Ludiomil / maprotiline	Sedating NE antidepressant. Peaks in 12 hours, half gone in 51 hours.
MAOI	A class of antidepressants that can be very effective but unfortunately require dietary restrictions. Eating the wrong food could potentially cause a stroke.
Maprotiline / **Ludiomil**	
Marijuana / cannabis	Increases dopamine 6 fold. Peaks in 20-30 minutes. May still be in body 28 days (positive urinanalysis).
Melatonin	Derived from serotonin and may help sleep in a dose of 3-6 mg; rarely as much as 20 mg is used. Can destabilize like an anti-depressant (page 38).
Mesoridazine / **Serentil**	
Methocarbamol / **Robaxin**	
Methylphenidate / **Ritalin**	
Metoprolol / **Lopressor, Toprol-XL**	Beta adrenergic blocker for palpitations. Half gone in 3-7 hours. See page 126.
Mellaril / thioridazine	Antipsychotic lowers dopamine, useful as a sleeper in 1-3% dose range. Peaks in 2 - 4 hours.

Moban / molindone

Antipsychotic that may also decrease weight. Tends to have more neurotoxic side effects in my practice.

Molindone / **Moban**

Morphine / opiate

Half gone in about 2 hours, highly addictive.

Naltrexone / **Trexan**

Nardil / phenelzine

MAOI antidepressant (stroke possible if dietary restrictions not followed).

Navane / thiothixene

Antipsychotic, potent, mildly sedating.

Nefazodone / **serzone**

Nicoderm

Each skin patch delivers nicotine for 24 hours to help smokers stop their habit. Less morning craving.

Nicorette

Nicotine chewing gum to help smokers stop over a 4-6 month period.

Nicotine / tobacco

A cigarette delivers 1-2 mg which peaks in 10-15 minutes and is half gone in 2 hours. Cancer risk is raised. Nicotine causes depression, irritability, and anxiety. Nicotine increases cholesterol. Silent heart attacks increase 3-fold in frequency, and 12-fold in duration.

Nicotrol

Each skin patch delivers nicotine for 16 hours to help smokers stop their habit. Less sleep disturbances.

Norpramine / desipramine

Potent activating tricyclic NE antidepressant, half gone in 22 hours

Nortriptyline / **Pamelar**

Orap / pimozide

An antipsychotic that is used for Tourette's disorder.

Oxazepam / **Serax**

Pamelar / nortriptyline

A NE / serotonin tricyclic antidepressant, half gone in 32 hours.

Parlodel / bromocriptine

For rigidity of Neuroleptic Malignant Syndrome (page 146).

Parnate / tranylcypromine

MAOI antidepressant (stroke possible if dietary restrictions not followed).

Paroxetine / **Paxil**

Paxil / paroxetine

A potent serotonin antidepressant (SSRI) that peaks in 5 hours and is half gone in 24 hours.

Pemoline / **Cylert**

Perphenazine / **Trilafon**

Phenelzine / **Nardil**

Phentermine resin / **Ionamin**

Phenytoin / **Dilantin**

Pimozide / **Orap**

Procyclidine / **Kemadrin**

Prolixin / fluphenazine   Nonsedating antipsychotic, peaks in 2-4 hours.

Propranolol / **Inderal**

Prostep   Each skin patch delivers nicotine for 24 hours to help smokers stop their habit. Less morning craving.

Protriptyline / **Vivactil**

Prozac / fluoxetine   A potent serotonin antidepressant (SSRI). Peaks in 7 hours, half out of body in 9 days.

Prosom / estazolam   Benzodiazepine GABA sleeper, peaks in 2 hours, half gone in 14 hours.

Quazepam / **Doral**

Restoril / temazepam   Benzodiazepine GABA sleeper, peaks in 1.5 hours, half gone in 13 hours.

Risperdal / risperidone   Nonsedating antipsychotic, few side effects.

Risperidone / **Risperdal**

Ritalin / methylphenidate   See amphetamine. Peaks in 1.9 hours and is half gone in 3 hours. Slow release form peaks in 4.7 hours, and lasts 8 hours.

Robaxin / methocarbamol   Muscle relaxer useful for cramping during heroin / opiate detox.

S-P-T   Thyroid medicine, mixture of T_4 and T_3 (2.5:1).

Serax / oxazepam   Calms anxiety by GABA enhancement (benzodiazepine). Peaks in 3 hours, half gone in 7 hours.

Serentil / mesoridazine   Similar to Mellaril, but injectable.

Sertraline / **Zoloft**

Serzone / nefazodone   An antidepressant related to Desyrel, but is not sedating, peaks in 1 hour and is half gone in 3 hours.

Sinequan / doxepin   Sedating antidepressant, half out in 17 hours.

SNRI   Selective norepinephrine serotonin reuptake inhibitor (NE / S antidepressant), Effexor.

SSRI   Selective serotonin reuptake inhibitor (serotonin antidepressant): Zoloft, Paxil, Prozac.

Stelazine / trifluoperazine

Potent nonsedating antipsychotic, peaks in 2-4 hours.

Surmontil / trimipramine

Antidepressant, sedating, half gone in 10 hours.

Symmetrel / amantadine

By increasing dopamine this decreases Parkinson's symptoms (see page 96), cocaine withdrawal craving and influenza A infections.

Synthroid / levothyroxine

Thyroid medicine (T_4) half gone in 6 days.

T_3

A more potent, sometimes destabilizing form of thyroid hormone.

T_4

A more physiologic (natural) form of thyroid hormone that tends to be gentler.

Taractan / chlorprothixene

Antipsychotic

Tegretal / carbamazepine

Stabilizes unstable electricity, moods and especially explosivity. Has a structure resembling an antidepressant (tricyclic). Peaks in 4-5 hours, half gone in 15 hours.

Temazepam / **Restoril**

Tenormin / atenolol

$Beta_1$ blocker that decreases palpitations, tremor and hypertension. It is safer than Inderal for patients with asthma, heart failure or diabetes. It peaks in 2-4 hours and is half gone in 7 hours.

Tenuate / diethylpropion

A diet pill that is a mild amphetamine and resembles structurally Wellbutrin. It can be useful for ADHD chemistry. Half gone in 6 hours.

Thioridazine / **Mellaril**

Thiothixene / **Navane**

Thorazine / chlorpromazine

A sedating antipsychotic.

Thyrar

Thyroid medicine mixture of T_4 and T_3 (7:1)

Thyrolar

Thyroid medicine mixture of T_4 and T_3 (4:1)

Tofranil / imipramine

A tricyclic antidepressant with a reputation for helping anxiety and insomnia. Peaks in 1.5 hours, half gone in 25 hours.

Tranxene / clorazepate

GABA enhancing benzodiazepine, peaks in 1-2 hours, half gone in 73 hours.

Tranylcypromine / **Parnate**

Trazadone / **Desyrel**

Trexan / naltrexone

Blocks the effects of opiates (heroin) to help prevent relapse in addicts.

Triazolam / **Halcion**

Tricylics	A group of antidepressants that can be effective, but are dangerous to overdose on. Some are sedating.
Trifluoperazine / **Stelazine**	
Trihexyphenidyl / **Artane**	
Trilafon / perphenazine	Antipsychotic.
Trimipramine / **Surmontil**	
Tyramine	Closely related to norepinephrine and epinephrine, this is a breakdown amino acid product of tyrosine. Patients on MAOI's cannot eat food containing this.
Tyrosine	An amino acid that is used to make thyroid hormone, dopamine, norepinephrine and epinephrine.
Urecholine / bethanechol	Stimulates the bladder to contract if urinary retention is occurring.
Valium / diazepam	Calms anxiety by GABA enhancement (benzodiazepine), peaks in 2 hours, half gone in 73 hours.
Valproic acid / **Depakote**	
Venlafaxine / **Effexor**	
Vistaril / hydroxyzine	A sedating antihistamine.
Vivactil / protriptyline	Antidepressant, activating, half gone in 78 hours.
Wellbutrin / bupropion	An antidepressant that structurally resembles a diet pill, and so is useful for adults with attention deficit disorder. It has seizure risk in high dose ranges. Peak is in 2 hours and it is half gone in 14 hours.
Xanax / alprazolam	Potent GABA enhancer (benzodiazepine) useful for calming anxiety and some depressions. Peaks in 1-2 hours, half gone in 11 hours.
Zoloft / sertraline	A potent serotonin antidepressant (SSRI) that peaks in 6 hours and is half gone in 26 hours.
Zolpidem / **Ambien**	

APPENDIX REFERENCES

TEXTBOOK REFERENCES   *** = Daily Use

1. *Advances in Psychopharmacology: Predicting and Improving Treatment Response* (1986)
   Gold, M.D./Lydiard, Ph.D.,M.D./Carman, M.D.

2. *Clinical Neurology for Psychiatrists* (1990), Kaufman   *

3. *Clinical Psychiatry and the Law, 2nd. Ed.*
   Robert Simon, M.D.

4. *Comprehensive Textbook of Psychiatry,* 7th Ed., 1994
   Harold Kaplan, M.D. and Benjamin Sadock, M.D.   **

5. *Current Medical Diagnosis and Treatment* (1994)
   Tierney, Jr., M.D./McPhee, M.D./Papadakis, M.D.   ***

6. *Drug Evaluations Annual 1994* - AMA   ***

7. DSM IV

8. *Family Medicine Principals and Practice,* 4th Ed. (1994)   *
   R. Taylor

9. *Handbook of Drug Therapy in Psychiatry, 2nd. Ed.* (1988)
   Jerrold Bernstein, M.D.

10. *Laboratory and Diagnostic Testing in Psychiatry* (1989)
    Rosse, M.D./Giese, M.D./Deutsch, M.D./Morihisa, M.D.

11. *Lithium Encyclopedia for Clinical Practice, 2nd. Ed.* (1987)   *
    Jefferson, M.D./Greist, M.D./Ackerman, M.S./Carroll, B.A.

12. *Manic Depressive Illness* (1990)
    Frederick Goodwin, M.D. and Kay Jamison, Ph.D.   *

13. *Manual of Clinical Problems in Psychiatry* (1990)
    Steven Hyman, M.D. and Michael Jenike, M.D.

14. *Manual of Clinical Psychopharmacology, 2nd. Ed.* (1991)
    Alan Schatzberg, M.D. and Jonathan Cole, M.D.

15. *The Medical Basis of Psychiatry, 2nd. Ed.* (1994)
    George Winokur, M.D. and Paula Clayton, M.D.

16. *The Molecular Foundations of Psychiatry* (1993)
    Steven Hyman, M.D. and Eric Nestler, M.D., Ph.D.

17. *The Pharmocological Basis of Therapeutics* (1993)
    Goodman, Gilman

18. *Physicians Desk Reference 1995*   ***

19. *Principals and Practice of Psychopharmacotherapy* (1993)
    Janicak, M.D./Davis, M.D./Preskorn, M.D./Ayd, Jr., M.D.

20. *Psychotropic Drugs Fast Facts* (1991)   **
    Jerrold Maxmen, M.D.

21. *Review of Psychiatry, Vol. 13* (1994)
    John Oldham, M.D. and Michelle Riba, M.D.

22. *Textbook of Medical Physiology* (1991)   *
    Guyton

REFERENCES - JOURNALS, OTHER

23. Rao, Gross, Strebel, Braunig, Huber, Klosterkotter, (Germany)
    Serum Amino Acids, Central Monoamines and Hormones in Drug Naive, Drug Free, and Neuroleptic treated Schizophrenic Patients and Healthy subjects.
    Psychiatry Research, 34:243-257 (1990)

24. McLarty, Ratcliff, Ratcliff, Shimmmins, Goldberg. *A Study of Thyroid Function in Psychiatric In-Patients.*
    British Journal of Psychiatry. 133:211-218 (1978)

25. Mark Gold, M.D., *Good News About Depression.* page 148 (1986)

26. Tejani-Butt, Yang; *A Time Course of Altered Thyroid States on the Noradrenergic System in Rat Brain by Quantitative Autoradiography.* Neuroendocrinology, 1994 March 59(3):235-44

27. Meites; *Role of Hypothalamic Catecholamines in Aging Process.*
    Acta Endocrinologica, 1991, 125 Suppl. 1:98-103

28. Upadhyaya, Agrawal; *Effect of L-Thyroxine and Carbimazole on Brain Biogenic Amines and Amino Acids in Rats.*
    Endocrine Research, 1993, 19(2-3):87-99

29. Weiss, Stein, Trommer, Refetoff; *Attention Deficit Disorder and Thyroid Function.*
    Journal of Pediatrics, 1993 Oct, 123(4):539-45

30. Raitiere, *Clinical Evidence for Thyroid Dysfunction in Patients with Seasonal Affective Disorder.*
    Psychoneuroendocrinology, 1992 May-July, 17(2-3):231-41

31. Cameron, Crocker; *The Hypothyroid Rat as a Model of Increased Sensitivity to Dopamine Receptor Agonists.* Pharmacology,
    Biochemistry and Behavior, 1990 Dec., 37(4):627-32

32. *Getting Stronger,* Bill Pearl, 1986

33. *Drugs and the Brain,* S. Snyder

REFERENCES FOR MEDICATION ACTIONS: [Graph on Page 20, Page 31]

1, 2: Antidepressants increase the availability of serotonin and norepinephrine - <u>Handbook of Drug Therapy in Psychiatry, 2nd edition, J. Bernstein (1988), page 127.</u>

3:　(a) Lithium stabilizes or **inhibits excess norepinephrine** (and dopamine). It enhances low serotonin (b) and thus **enhances low NE** since these systems interact. This was a difficult, hopefully realistic, and approximate extrapolation from complex theory in:
　　(a) <u>The Pharmacological Basis of Therapeutics,</u>
　　　　Goodman/Gilman, 1993, page 418.
　　 (b) <u>APA Annual Review,</u> 1985, page 45.

4:　Anticonvulsants stabilize excessive discharge by neurons notably those that are electrical. For example, extremely unstable electricity causes seizures. <u>AMA Drug Evaluations,</u> (1994) pages 146, 365. Mild electrical instability may cause mood problems.

5:　Antipsychotics work by blocking brain dopamine receptors. <u>Principals and Practice of Psychopharmacotherapy,</u> Janicak, Davis, Preskorn, Ayd (1993), page 94.

6:　Attention deficit hyperactivity disorder is due to a deficiency in norepinephrine (or one of its precursors). <u>Comprehensive Textbook of Psychiatry IV,</u> Kaplan, Sadock (1985), page 1685. Dopamine and norepinephrine systems are involved. Low blood perfusion occurs in several brain areas of ADHD patients and is reversed with Ritalin (<u>The Molecular Foundations of Psychiatry,</u> (1993) Hyman MD, Nestler MD, PhD, page 294). The stimulants that structurally resemble DA/NE are best in treating ADHD. Thus the concept "DA/NE replacement treatment" is logical.

7:　Benzodiazapines facilitate (increase) the effects of GABA. <u>The Molecular Foundations of Psychiatry,</u> Hyman, Nestler, (1993) page 150.

8:　Beta adrenergic blockers block the action of catecholamines (dopamine, norepinephrine, epinephrine). Adrenaline is epinephrine. <u>The Pharmacologic Basis of Therapeutics,</u> Goodman/Gilman, 1993

9:　Thyroid profoundly effects to increase metabolic rate of the body. <u>Textbook of Medical Physiology,</u> Guyton (1991), page 831.

10: Estrogen may improve psychological symptoms in females. <u>Family Medicine, Principals and Practice,</u> 4th Ed., 1994, David, Johnson, Phillips, Scherger.